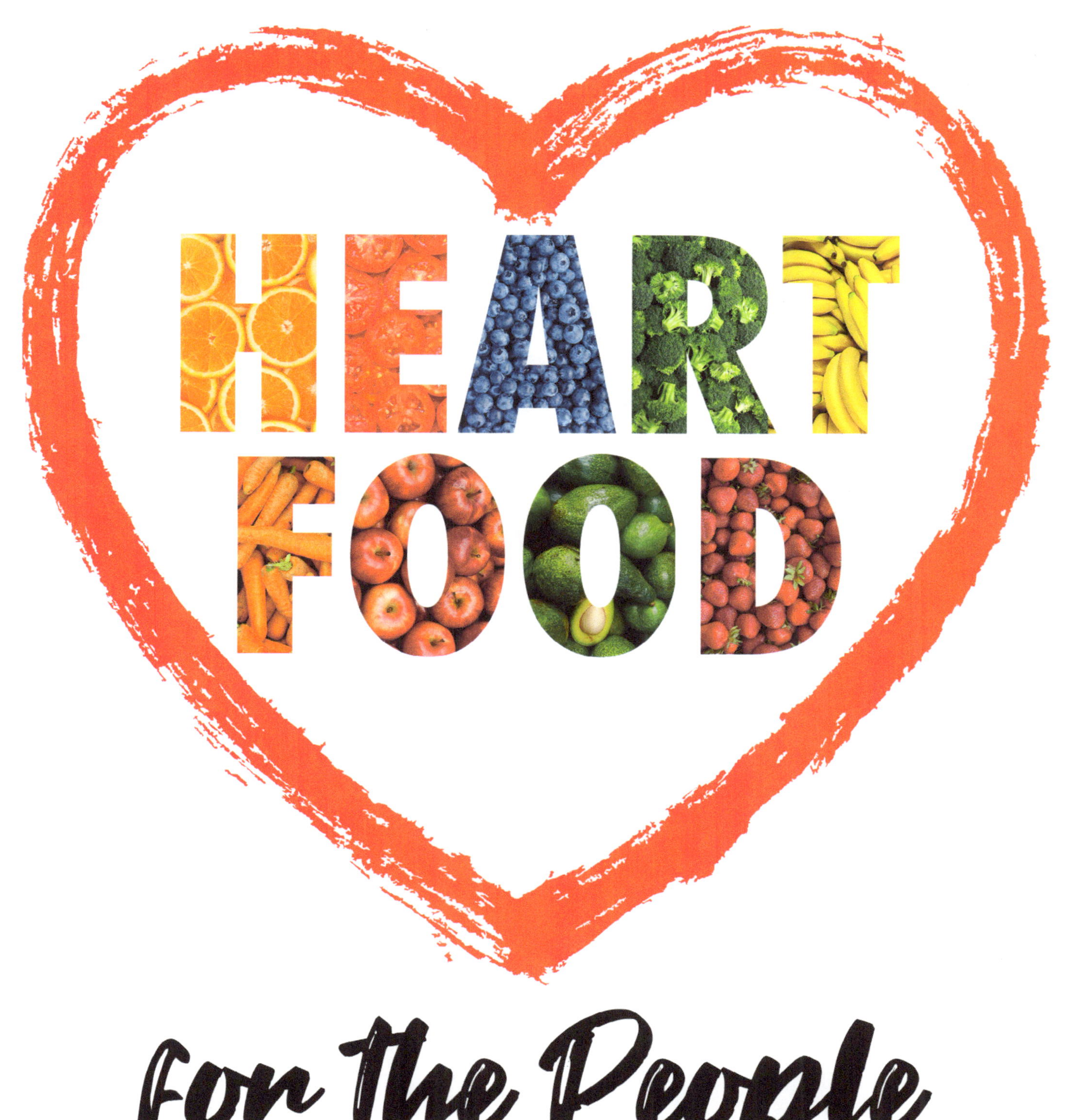

HEART
FOOD
for the People
A CARDIOLOGIST'S GUIDE TO HEALTH EMPOWERMENT
BREDY PIERRE-LOUIS, MD, FACC

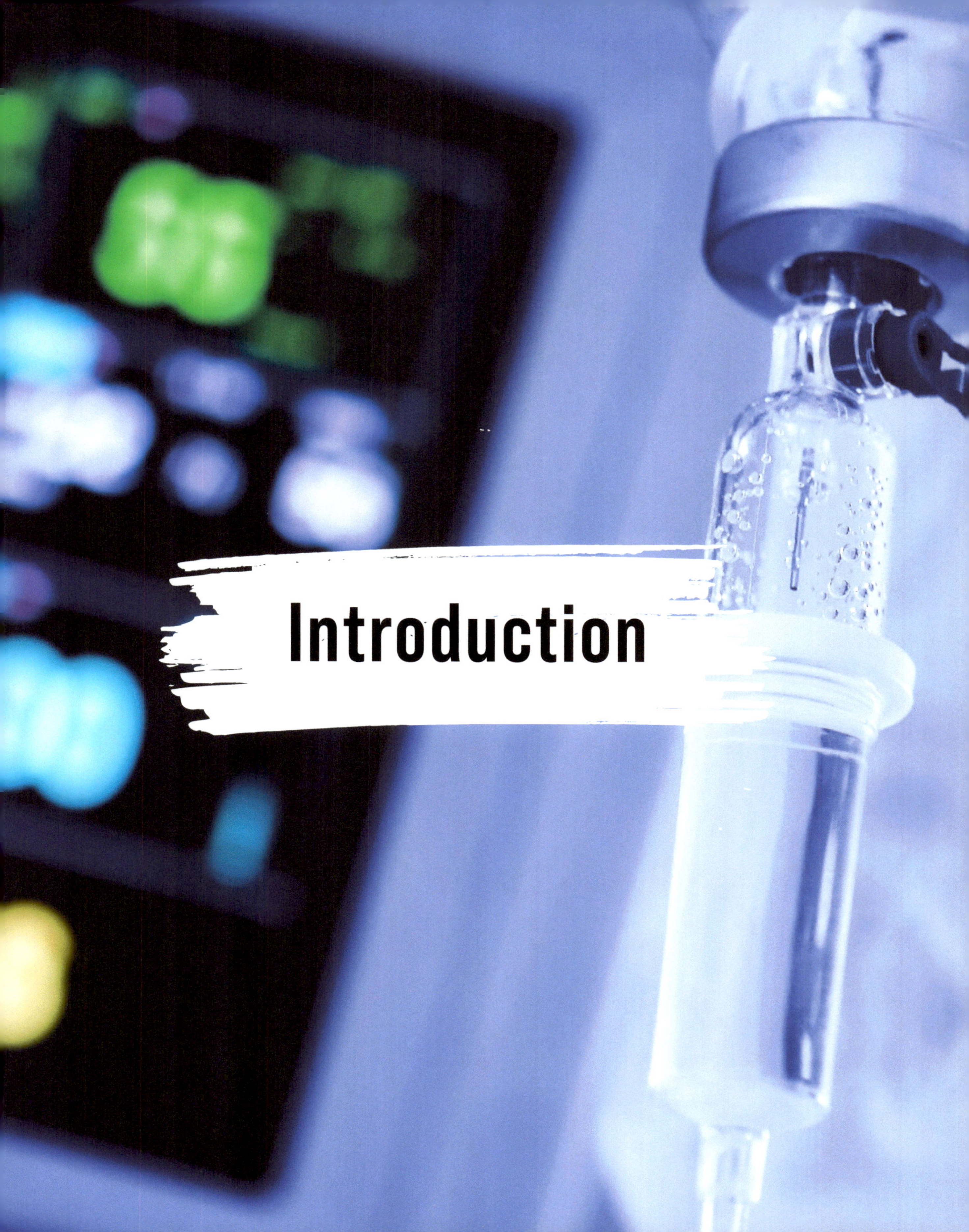

Introduction

INTRODUCTION

"Of all the forms of inequality, injustice in healthcare is the most shocking and inhumane."

– MARTIN LUTHER KING, JR.

Every 40 seconds a person in the United States will have a myocardial infarction (heart attack), approximately 805,000 each year. And every 40 seconds a person in the United States will have a cerebral infarction (stroke), approximately 795,000 each year. Over 900,000 people in the United States die annually from cardiovascular diseases, making them the leading causes of death, accounting for 1 of every 3 mortalities.

However, cardiovascular diseases do not have to be a fatal diagnosis. Clinical research studies estimate that over 90% of cardiovascular diseases can be prevented when patients have access to essential health and wellness resources.

Tragically, our healthcare system is in an escalating state of crisis, failing to support all patients in their journeys toward optimal health. Despite innovative new prevention protocols, medical therapeutics, diagnostic modalities, and minimally invasive interventions, over half the population in the United States is afflicted with the rising epidemics of hypertension, diabetes, dyslipidemia (abnormal cholesterol), obesity, and nicotine dependence — chronic conditions and risk factors that lead to cardiovascular diseases when left unmanaged.

Of primary concern is the cardiovascular health of patients in underserved communities, where access to nutritious food, open spaces to exercise, and preventive healthcare services is severely limited. Residents in these communities experience food insecurity, foodh deserts, excessive promotion of unhealthy ultra-processed (junk, fast) foods and nicotine products, and reduced access to quality medical care, all of which lead to an unequal incidence and prevalence of cardiovascular diseases. According to recent national data, patients in underserved communities experience a 30% increased risk of mortality from cardiovascular diseases compared to patients in better-resourced communities. This represents an extremely significant disparity of morbidity and results in dramatically reduced life expectancy, including death 15 years prematurely for the most vulnerable underserved communities. As a result of these lethal healthcare disparities and inequities in the United States, underserved communities suffer millions of lost years of life every decade.

Health disparities and inequities are the devastating consequences of historical and current economic, political, social, and environmental injustices entrenched in our healthcare system and society, including structural racism, generational poverty, and residential segregation. These social determinants of health severely impact the lives of underserved communities, precluding us from achieving our full physical and mental potential, and significantly limiting our longevity. Health inequity can only be overcome through radical and revolutionary changes in our medical system, including universal single-payer healthcare, expansion of community-based healthcare centers in every population, and a publicly subsidized focus on preventive health for every community. Health activists, progressive healthcare providers, and grassroots organizations are fiercely engaged in this important struggle, and we must all contribute to this vital movement to ensure their efforts and sacrifices achieve equity for everyone.

UNDERSERVED COMMUNITIES

Underserved communities are *the People* experiencing significant health disparities and inequities because of historical and current economic, political, social, and environmental injustices:

1. Financially under-resourced and economically disadvantaged communities and households, including the working class and people struggling with poverty, experience limited access to quality, timely medical care and endure significant healthcare disparities

2. Black, Indigenous, Latino, and Asian and Pacific Islander communities are underserved and experience healthcare disparities independent of income

3. Collectively, underserved communities represent more than 75% of the United States population

A STRATEGY FOR THE UNDERSERVED

Until we implement fundamental changes and transform healthcare into a truly guaranteed basic human right, underserved communities need our own evidence-based strategy to preserve our health and protect our lives.

This patient-inspired book, HEART FOOD *for the People*, introduces this strategy — **Health Empowerment** — and provides guidance for the millions of people who lack the direct support they need to lead the healthiest lives possible.

HEALTH EMPOWERMENT

Health Empowerment is the lifelong process of maximizing your potential for wellness, independent of the healthcare system.

It involves self-directed, health-promoting behaviors that focus on nutritious food, regular exercise, and disease prevention strategies.

The Health Empowerment strategy is based on extensive clinical research that proves you can reduce your risk of cardiovascular diseases, and the chronic conditions that cause them, by implementing healthy lifestyle choices. When you make the change to heart-healthy nutrition, exercise regularly, and prioritize prevention and wellness, you empower yourself to live a longer life in good health.

Start your Health Empowerment strategy by reading HEART FOOD *for the People* in its entirety several times, and then, beginning with the aspects that resonate with you most, progressively implement all of the recommendations in every section. During your personal journey to optimal health always use this guide as an essential resource.

We encourage you to make changes on your own timetable. To help you succeed, we offer recommendations for introducing a new way of eating and healthier behaviors at different paces: gradual, slow, moderate, or immediate.

Your path to better health begins now. Implement the Health Empowerment strategy starting today, and you will live longer and live better.

HEART FOOD *for the People!*

Bredy Pierre-Louis, MD, FACC is a board-certified cardiologist currently practicing in New York who has been working to empower underserved communities for over 25 years.

HOW TO USE THIS RESOURCE

Changing health behaviors is very challenging, especially given the deep-rooted obstacles imposed by societal injustices. But Health Empowerment is a necessary reality to ensure the wellness of everyone in our communities.

We must make a change now, and this book addresses the challenges underserved communities face to embrace Health Empowerment. It offers evidence-based strategies, basic recommendations, and empowering resources that will help you and your family achieve wellness, prevent cardiovascular diseases, and overcome the disparities in our healthcare system that affect your right to a long life free of preventable diseases.

The Health Empowerment strategy is outlined in seven sections:

1. **A DETAILED NUTRIENT GLOSSARY** and a focused description of cardiovascular disease mechanisms to ensure you understand the basic and essential elements of a heart-healthy diet and how each food and nutrient you eat promotes wellness and prevents cardiovascular diseases.

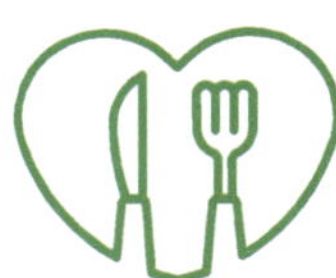

2. **HEART-HEALTHY SNACKS AND HEALTHIER FOOD OPTIONS** to eliminate unhealthy food items and ensure everything you eat and drink will make you live longer and live better.

3. **A DETAILED SHOPPING LIST** of heart-healthy foods and beverages every person should include in their diet. We understand the limitations imposed by food deserts, where nutritious and healthy foods are hard to find. Therefore, we have included food options that are available in traditionally underserved communities.

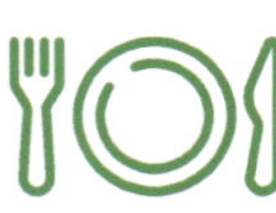

4. **A DETAILED 3-MEAL-A-DAY FOOD PLAN FOR 7 DAYS**, presented in an easy-to-follow format that gives you **21 separate healthy meals plus healthy snacks** you can implement immediately, with explanations of why each food is heart-healthy.

5. **A PLAN FOR INTEGRATING EXERCISE INTO YOUR HEALTH BEHAVIORS** and resources for implementing additional heart-healthy alterations to your lifestyle.

6. **A STRUCTURED PLAN FOR MONITORING YOUR RISK FACTORS** to optimize your Health Empowerment strategy, promote wellness, and prevent cardiovascular diseases.

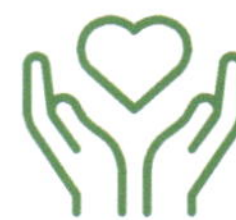

7. **A STRATEGY TO TRANSFORM YOUR PERSONAL JOURNEY TO OPTIMAL HEALTH** into a movement that advocates for equity, makes meaningful change, and creates a reality where healthcare is a truly guaranteed basic human right for everyone.

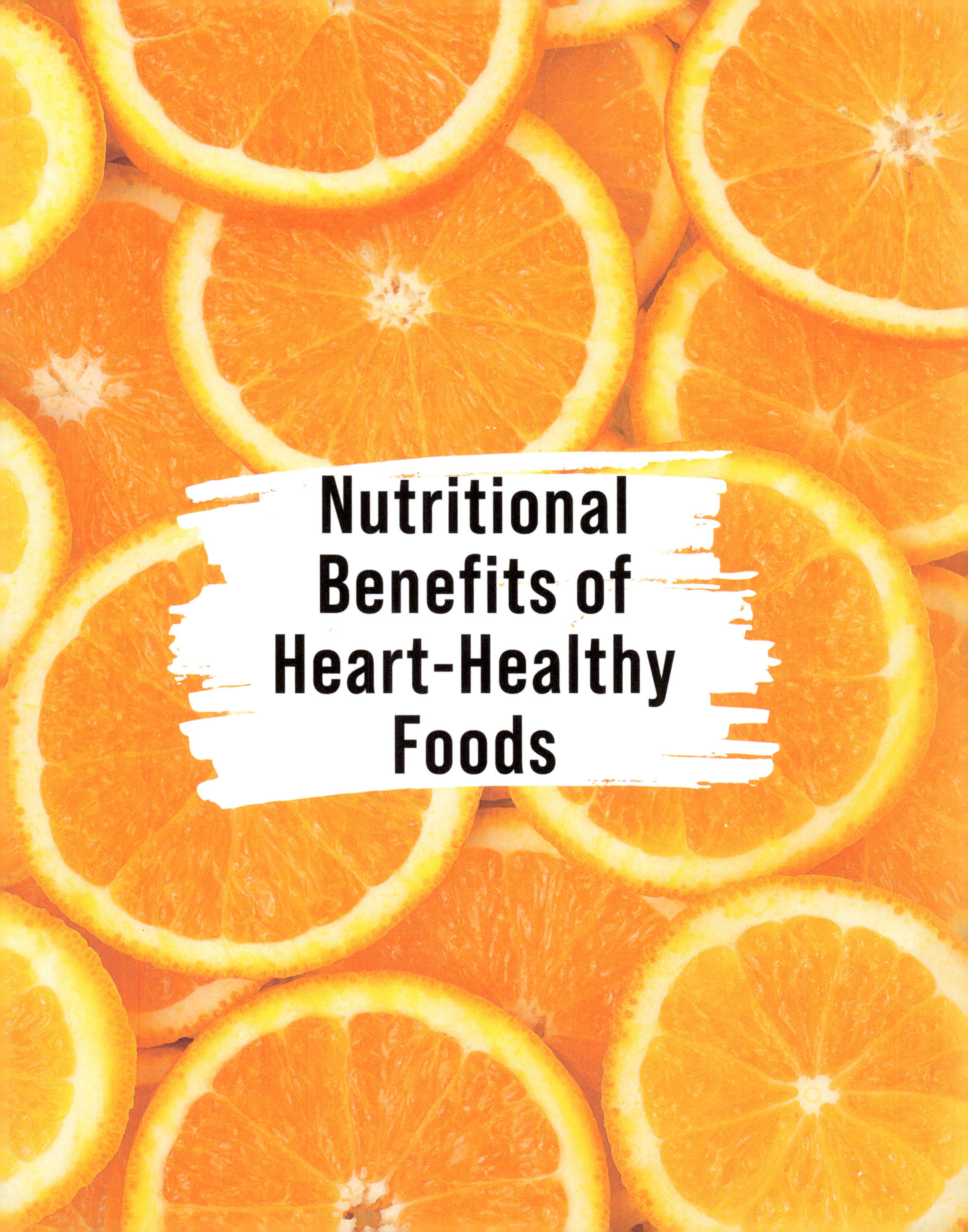

Nutritional
Benefits of
Heart-Healthy
Foods

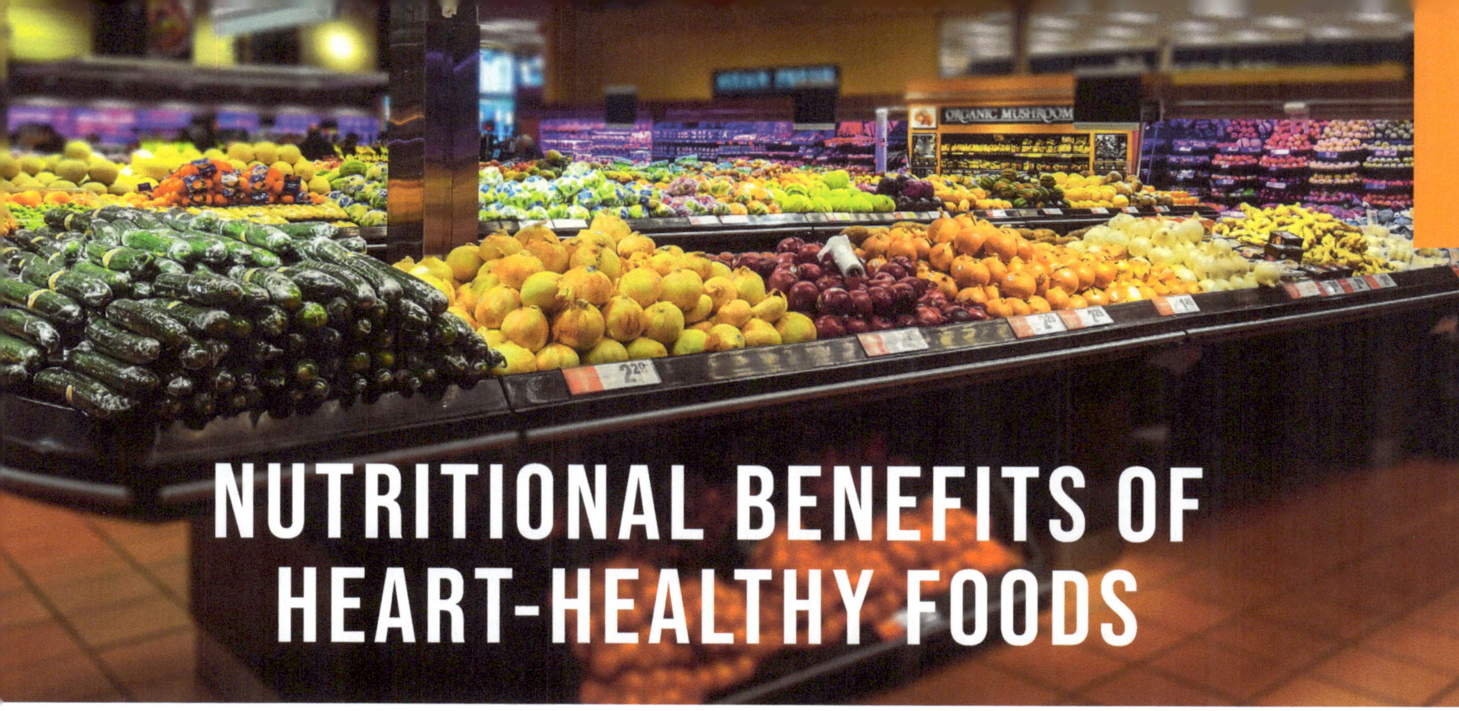

NUTRITIONAL BENEFITS OF HEART-HEALTHY FOODS

Preventable cardiovascular diseases, including myocardial and cerebral infarctions (heart attacks and strokes), are the result of damage and injury to the arteries and blood vessels (vascular damage/injury) that circulate blood and oxygen to vital organs and tissues in the body. This vascular damage and injury, known as atherosclerosis, is an inflammatory disease commonly described as a buildup of plaque along the artery walls. Progressive plaque buildup results in obstructive blood clots or ruptured arteries that deprive the heart and brain of oxygen.

Atherosclerosis is initiated by oxygen free radicals, which are unstable molecules produced by biochemical reactions in the body, that can damage or alter the structure of cells. Vascular damage and injury caused by oxygen free radicals allow low-density lipoprotein LDL (bad) cholesterol to deposit along the inside of artery walls, contributing to the development of plaque in the arteries. The body uses antioxidants that it produces and extracts from certain foods to neutralize oxygen free radicals. However, an imbalance between the production of oxygen free radicals and the body's ability to eliminate them creates a condition called oxidative stress. Oxidative stress increases the progression of atherosclerosis.

Basic science and clinical research studies have proven that a heart-healthy diet with an optimal balance of macro and micronutrients (along with cardiac exercise and nicotine cessation) reduces inflammation, oxygen free radicals, oxidative stress, and LDL (bad) cholesterol levels. When initiated early, a heart-healthy diet also helps prevent hypertension, diabetes, dyslipidemia (abnormal cholesterol), and obesity — recognized risk factors that accelerate atherosclerosis and the onset of cardiovascular diseases.

In fact, a heart-healthy diet is the most effective strategy for maintaining healthy arteries and blood vessels and preventing vascular damage and injury.

And it is an empowering change we can implement independently of the healthcare system.

When we adopt a heart-healthy diet, we will not only prevent atherosclerosis and cardiovascular diseases. Because the inflammatory disease process is also involved in non-cardiac diseases, including many cancers, the Health Empowerment strategy promotes overall wellness and helps everyone live longer and better.

We believe that when you understand the specific nutrients in a heart-healthy diet that prevent cardiovascular diseases, you will feel more empowered to incorporate these foods into your nutrition plan. Therefore, we have included a glossary of the macro and micronutrients that are too often lacking in the diets of underserved communities because of limited availability and awareness.

We discuss these nutrients again in our individual meal plans, along with further descriptions of their benefits and explanations about why they are essential for your health, to ensure you understand and feel confident that all the food you eat is heart-healthy and contributes to your complete wellness.

MACRONUTRIENTS

Macronutrients are the four major food groups your body requires in large amounts (grams) to function properly.

Lean (Low-Fat) Protein

Protein is a nutrient composed of amino acids your body uses to grow and maintain cells. Protein exists in every cell of your body, including your organs, muscles, bones, and even your skin, nails, and hair.

But your body cannot store excess protein, it either uses it for energy or stores it as fat. Therefore, you need to supply your body with healthy, lean protein from the food you eat daily.

Without protein, your body cannot build and repair muscle and tissue or create the enzymes you need to digest your food. When you do not consume enough lean protein, you lose energy, and your heart and respiratory systems are compromised. You need different amounts of lean protein depending on your age and activity level.

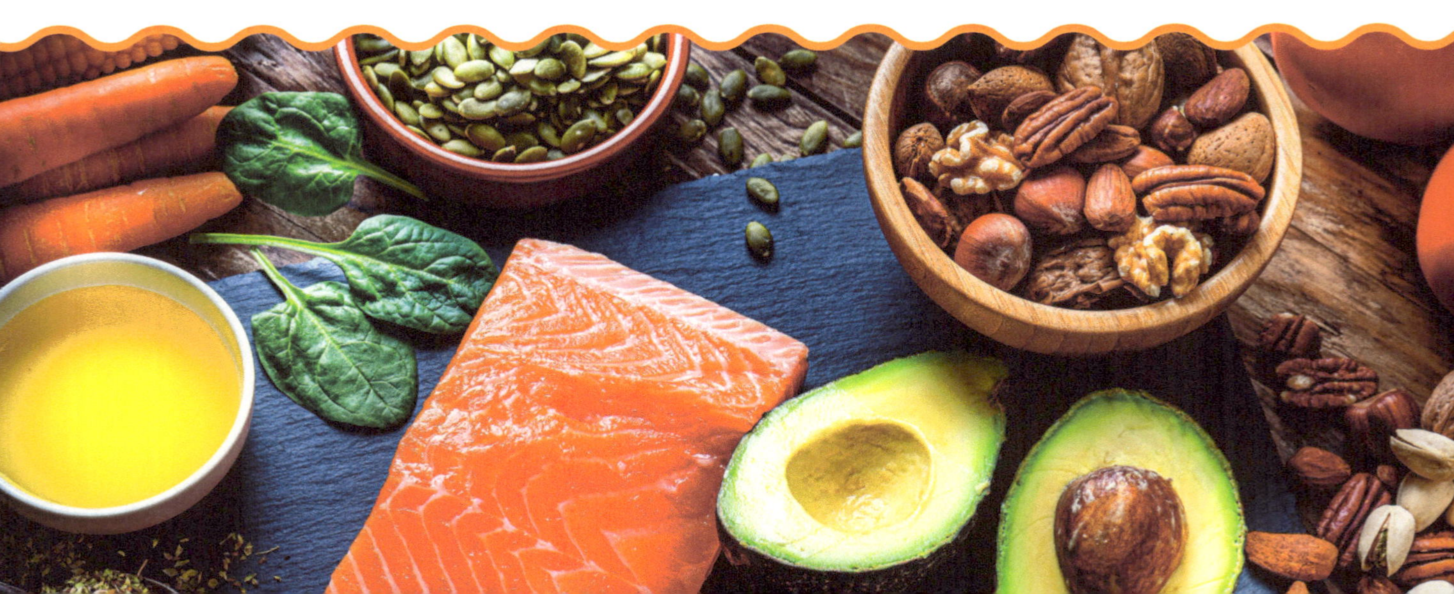

Sources of healthy, lean protein include beans, nuts, fish, and skinless chicken breast.

Unsaturated Fat

Unsaturated fats help proteins function properly and maintain cell health. Fat also helps your body absorb fat-soluble vitamins, such as vitamins A, D, and E.

The foods we consume contain either good fats or bad fats.

Unsaturated fats are good fats because they increase your high-density lipoprotein HDL (good) cholesterol and decrease your low-density lipoprotein LDL (bad) cholesterol, preventing vascular damage and injury, atherosclerosis, and cardiovascular diseases. They also help reduce systemic inflammation in your body.

Sources of unsaturated fats include fish and plant-based foods like vegetables, nuts, and olive oil.

There are two types of unsaturated fats, monounsaturated and polyunsaturated:

- monounsaturated fats are found in olive oil, avocados, and nuts
- polyunsaturated fats, including essential omega-3 fatty acids, are found in fish

Saturated fats, the bad fats (including extremely unhealthy trans fats), come from animal-based foods, including beef, pork, certain cuts of chicken (skin, thighs, legs, wings), turkey, eggs, dairy products (all cow's milk, cheese, butter), shellfish (shrimp, clams, scallops, crab, lobster) and processed/ultra-processed foods (potato chips, ice cream, cookies, donuts). These foods raise your LDL (bad) cholesterol level. Therefore, consuming excessive amounts of saturated fats leads to vascular damage and injury and an increased risk of atherosclerosis and cardiovascular diseases.

Complex Carbohydrates

Carbohydrates provide the energy your body needs to sustain your organs, cells, and tissues. Carbohydrates break down into glucose (simple sugar) in your digestive tract. Different types of carbohydrates release different amounts of glucose into your bloodstream.

We measure how much a carbohydrate increases your blood glucose levels with the glycemic index. Simple carbohydrates (known as sugars) like cane sugar, fructose, lactose, and sucrose are high on the glycemic index and raise your blood glucose levels quickly. Refined carbohydrates, including white bread, white rice, and non-whole wheat pasta, have important nutrients removed and are also high on the glycemic index. Simple and refined carbohydrates increase the risk of developing diabetes, obesity, and cardiovascular diseases.

Complex carbohydrates are low on the glycemic index and break down more slowly, providing your body with a more lasting source of energy. Complex carbohydrates also contain fiber which helps with digestion, promotes healthy gut bacteria in your digestive tract, and helps your body absorb important nutrients.

Sources of complex carbohydrates include oatmeal, whole grain wheat and bran cereals, granola, brown rice, and sweet potatoes.

Fiber

A heart-healthy diet requires sufficient daily fiber, yet the current average consumption is approximately half the recommended allowance. Clinical research studies have demonstrated that people who eat more fiber are significantly less likely to develop cardiovascular diseases. Fiber has been shown to lower LDL (bad) cholesterol, reduce blood glucose, lower blood pressure, and help maintain a healthy weight. Therefore, fiber helps to prevent atherosclerosis, diabetes, hypertension, and obesity, which reduces the risk of cardiovascular diseases.

Fiber is a carbohydrate found in plant-based foods and does not break down during digestion, therefore it slows the food transit time from the stomach to the intestine, which makes you feel fuller for longer, thus limiting your caloric intake and preventing obesity.

Fiber also promotes healthy gut bacteria and intestinal health which reduces systemic inflammation that contributes to vascular damage and injury.

Sources of fiber include beans, oatmeal, whole grain wheat and bran cereals, granola, nuts, and fruits and vegetables including broccoli, carrots, tomatoes, apples, raspberries, blueberries, and oranges.

MICRONUTRIENTS

Micronutrients are the groups of vitamins, minerals, and antioxidants your body requires in small amounts (milligrams, micrograms) to function properly and stay healthy.

Fruits, vegetables, beans, oatmeal, whole grain wheat and bran cereals, and nuts are the primary sources of vitamins, minerals, and antioxidants.

Vitamins

Vitamins are essential nutrients that facilitate biochemical reactions in your body and promote good health. When you eat a heart-healthy diet, you provide your body with the vitamins it needs to promote wellness and prevent cardiovascular diseases:

- **VITAMIN A** is converted from carotenoids, the pigments in plants that give vegetables and fruits their color. Common carotenoids include beta-carotene, lutein, and lycopene. Carotenoids are antioxidants that remove oxygen free radicals, reduce oxidative stress, and limit vascular damage and injury. Vitamin A also helps lower your LDL (bad) cholesterol levels.
- **VITAMIN B-COMPLEX** includes the vitamins B1, B2, niacin, B5, B6, folic acid, and B12. These vitamins reduce

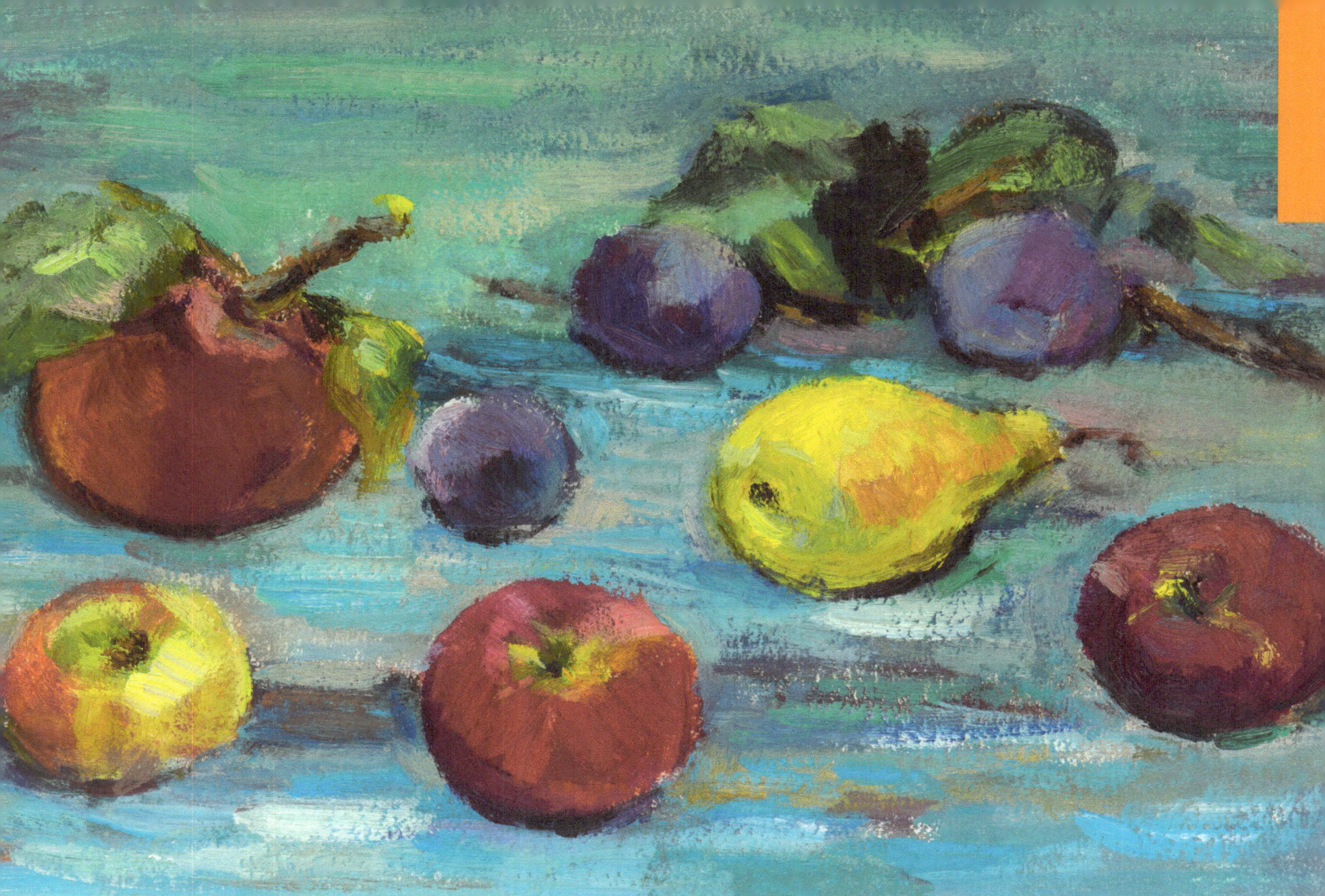

homocysteine levels. Homocysteine is an amino acid that increases the risk of cardiovascular diseases when elevated. B-complex vitamins also have significant antioxidant properties and prevent anemia.

- **VITAMIN C** is another strong antioxidant that reduces vascular inflammation, damage, and injury. It also lowers blood pressure and helps to prevent hypertension.

- **VITAMIN D** contributes to maintaining the proper levels of calcium and phosphorous and helps reduce blood pressure. Your body requires adequate sunlight exposure to make vitamin D.

- **VITAMIN E** is a powerful antioxidant that helps support vitamin A, together these vitamins can significantly reduce vascular inflammation, damage, and injury.

Minerals

Minerals are essential nutrients that facilitate biochemical reactions in your body and promote good health. Your body needs certain minerals to function properly. You improve your health and prevent cardiovascular diseases when you eat foods rich in the following minerals:

- **CALCIUM (CA)** is essential to normal cardiac and vascular function and helps reduce blood pressure.
- **COPPER (CU)** maintains a healthy metabolism and is especially important for the cardiovascular system. In conjunction with specific proteins, it functions as an antioxidant and prevents vascular damage and injury.
- **IRON (FE)** helps the body form hemoglobin, which transports oxygen in the blood to vital organs including the heart and brain. Iron deficiency leads to anemia, which increases the risk of vascular damage and injury.
- **MANGANESE (MN)** helps metabolize protein, carbohydrates, and cholesterol, which maintains healthy blood flow and prevents diabetes and atherosclerosis, it also has antioxidant properties that reduce inflammation and vascular damage and injury.
- **MAGNESIUM (MG)** activates enzymes needed to keep metabolism functioning properly and helps reduce blood pressure and LDL (bad) cholesterol.
- **PHOSPHORUS (P)** has antioxidant properties that reduce inflammation and vascular damage and injury.
- **POTASSIUM (K)** helps maintain proper water and electrolyte balance in your body. Adequate potassium levels help reduce blood pressure and reduce the risk of cardiovascular diseases.

Antioxidants

Antioxidants are nutrient compounds found in specific foods that neutralize and eliminate oxygen free radicals, reduce oxidative stress, and prevent vascular inflammation, damage, and injury. Many vitamins and minerals are natural antioxidants. A diet with a high concentration of antioxidants has been shown to prevent atherosclerosis and cardiovascular diseases.

PHYTONUTRIENTS are natural compounds that give edible plants their color, flavor, and smell, they have antioxidant properties that help prevent oxidative stress and reduce the risk of cardiovascular diseases. These antioxidants include **Resveratrol** which improves vascular function, maintains healthy blood flow, and reduces oxidative stress and inflammation, preventing the development of vascular damage and injury. Red grapes, apples, and blueberries are excellent sources of Phytonutrients.

POLYPHENOLS are natural chemical compounds found in plants. These antioxidants, including **Carvacrol and Oleocanthal**, improve vascular function, reduce inflammation, increase HDL (good) cholesterol, and decrease LDL (bad) cholesterol. Blueberries, apples, walnuts, almonds, spinach, carrots, chickpeas, oregano, and extra-virgin olive oil are excellent sources of Polyphenols.

FLAVONOIDS are a type of polyphenol found in many fruits and vegetables with bright colors. They improve vascular function, which is important for maintaining healthy blood flow. Flavonoids have also been shown to help reduce oxidative stress and inflammation that contribute to the development of cardiovascular diseases. **Anthocyanins** are a type of flavonoid that protects cells from damage by oxygen free radicals. **Quercetin** is another common flavonoid. These antioxidants give fruits and vegetables their red, blue, and purple colors. Blueberries, strawberries, and red onions are excellent sources of Flavonoids.

CAROTENOIDS, INCLUDING BETA-CAROTENE, are a type of pigment that gives many fruits and vegetables their color. With powerful antioxidant properties, they improve vascular function which is important for maintaining healthy blood flow. Carotenoids have also been shown to help reduce oxidative stress and inflammation, which can contribute to the development of cardiovascular diseases. **Lutein** is a type of carotenoid that gives plants their green color and is found in broccoli. **Lycopene** is a carotenoid that gives plants their red or pink color. Tomatoes are a great source of Lycopene. Carrots and sweet potatoes are also excellent sources of Carotenoids.

ALLICIN is a potent antioxidant found primarily in raw chopped or minced garlic that gives this vegetable its characteristic smell, it degrades with cooking therefore the benefits are derived from consuming raw garlic as part of a salad or using garlic powder as a condiment. This powerful antioxidant improves vascular function, removes oxygen free radicals, reduces oxidative stress and inflammation, and reduces LDL (bad) cholesterol, blood glucose, and blood pressure. Allicin also enhances the function of other natural antioxidants in the body and therefore has an amplifying effect to prevent cardiovascular diseases.

PROBIOTICS are live bacteria and yeast found in yogurt that help maintain a healthy balance of gut organisms which is essential for the optimal digestion of macro and micronutrients. Studies have demonstrated that consuming probiotics lowers LDL (bad) cholesterol, blood glucose, blood pressure, and body weight, and therefore helps prevent cardiovascular diseases. In addition, probiotics have antioxidant properties that reduce systemic inflammation which contributes to vascular damage and injury.

ACETIC ACID is the main organic compound found in vinegar and is responsible for both its unique flavor and acidity. It has several demonstrated benefits that help prevent cardiovascular diseases including its ability to lower blood pressure, blood glucose, LDL (bad) cholesterol, and body weight. In both red wine and apple cider vinegar acetic acid also functions as an antioxidant by reducing oxygen free radicals and oxidative stress which prevents vascular inflammation, damage, and injury leading to a reduced risk of cardiovascular diseases.

PIPERINE is an alkaloid compound and phytochemical responsible for the distinct flavor of black pepper and a strong antioxidant that improves vascular function, removes oxygen free radicals from the body, and reduces oxidative stress and inflammation. In addition, Piperine has a positive effect on macronutrient and micronutrient absorption which enhances the availability of other heart-healthy foods that help prevent cardiovascular diseases.

CAPSAICIN is a plant compound responsible for the heat flavor of cayenne peppers and a powerful antioxidant that improves vascular function, removes oxygen free radicals from the body, and reduces oxidative stress and inflammation. In addition, Capsaicin can increase the rate of fat metabolism which lowers LDL (bad) cholesterol and body weight and therefore helps prevent atherosclerosis and obesity.

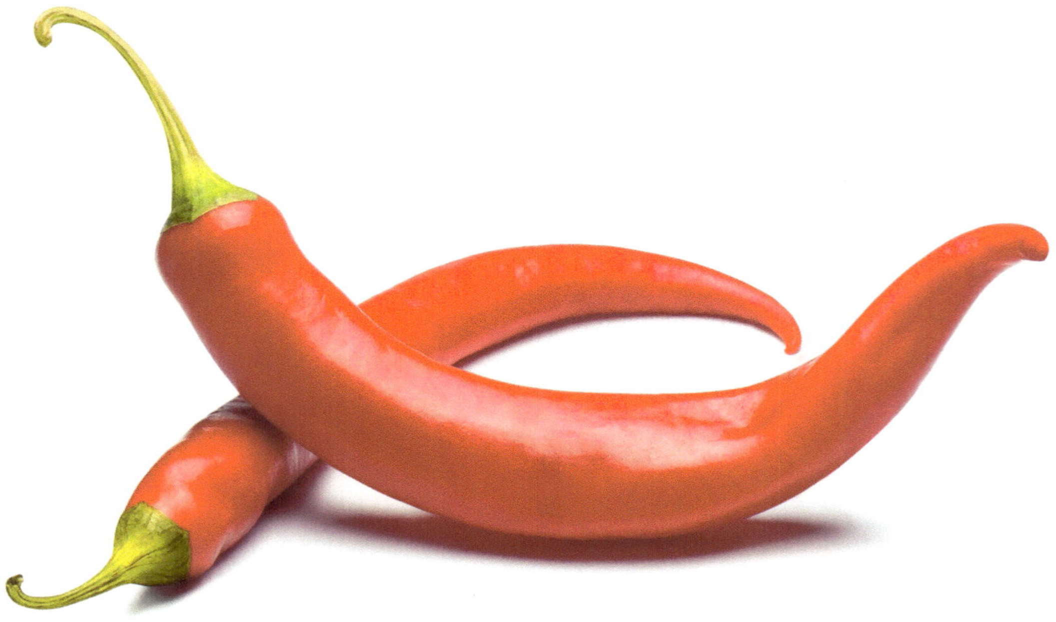

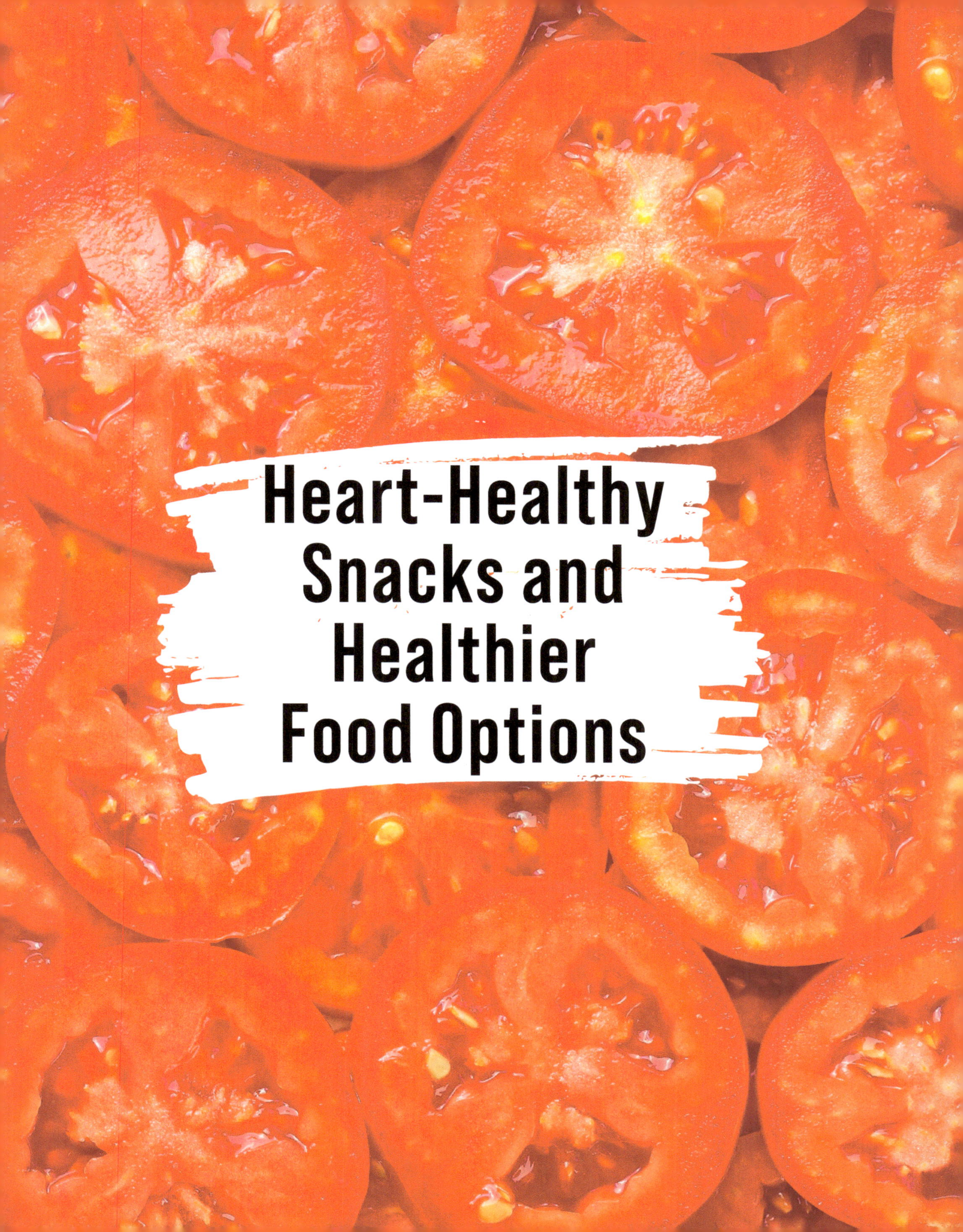
Heart-Healthy
Snacks and
Healthier
Food Options

HEART-HEALTHY SNACKS AND HEALTHIER FOOD OPTIONS

Eating between main meals is often unavoidable. Unfortunately, unhealthy snacking can add significant amounts of excessive processed sugar, salt, and saturated fat to your daily food intake, which increases your risk of cardiovascular diseases.

To consistently promote wellness, minimize the food you eat outside of the 21-meal plan, which includes heart-healthy snacks. Because the Health Empowerment nutrition strategy contains the recommended daily allowances for lean protein, complex carbohydrates, unsaturated fats, and fiber, it will ideally provide sufficient calories to prevent eating unhealthy snacks between meals. When you need a snack to sustain your energy, choose from the healthy foods in the 21-meal plan.

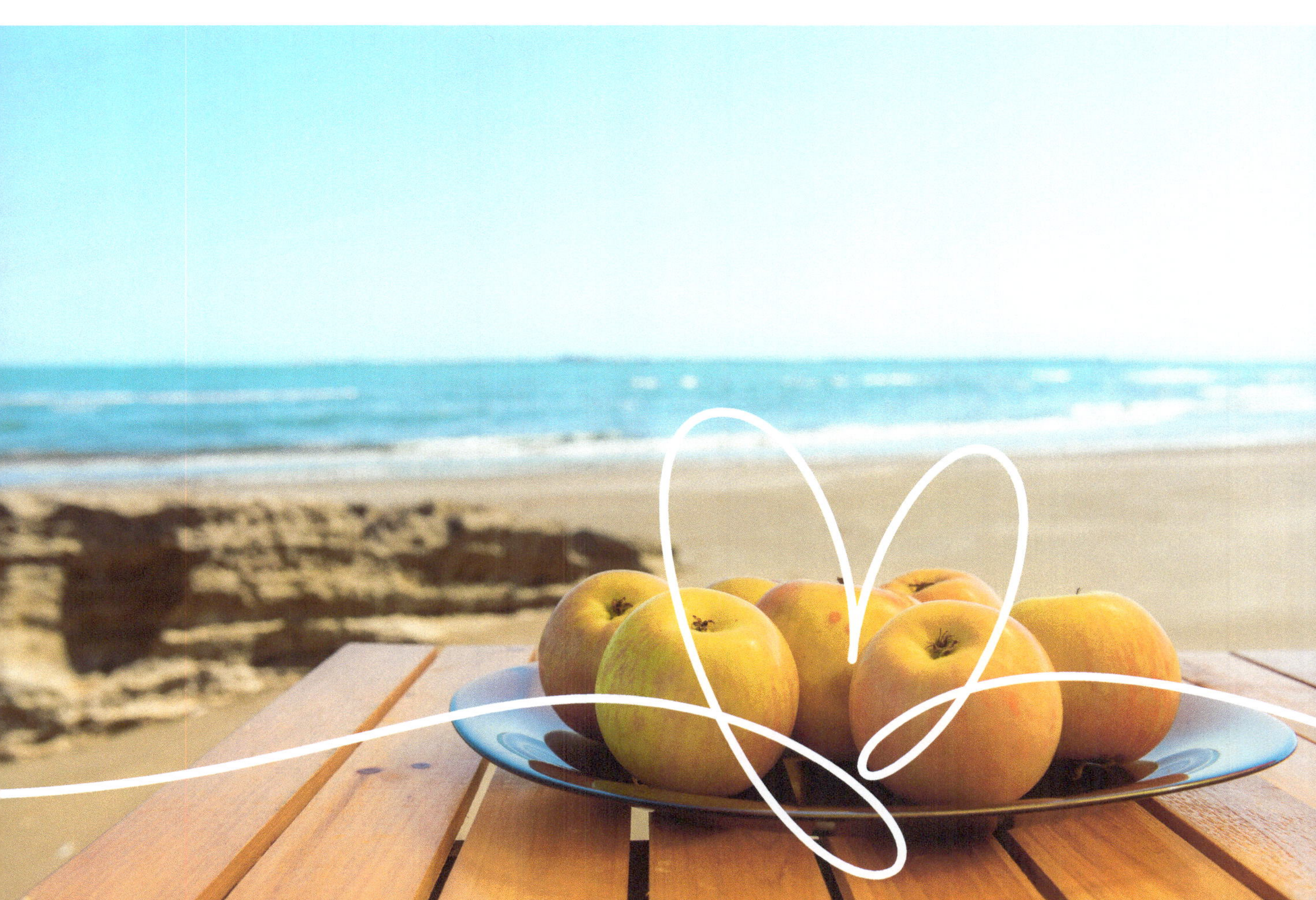

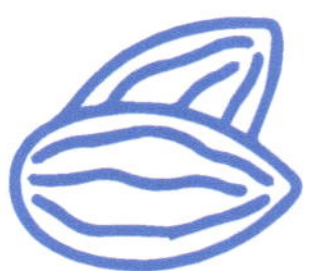

Nuts are high in lean protein, fiber, healthy unsaturated fats, and antioxidants. They contain most of the vitamins and minerals your body needs, making them an excellent snack when you are feeling depleted. Eating nuts four times a week is associated with a reduction in cardiovascular diseases including myocardial and cerebral infarctions (heart attacks and strokes).

When buying nuts, select options that have no added salt and no added sugar/honey. Check the ingredients label on the package under "Sodium" and "Carbohydrates" to confirm there is no added salt or sugar/honey.

WALNUTS: Walnuts are rich in copper, an antioxidant mineral that reduces oxygen free radicals and oxidative stress, and protects against vascular damage and injury. They also contribute manganese, magnesium, and unsaturated fats, which help reduce blood pressure and LDL (bad) cholesterol, making them very healthy for your heart.

ALMONDS: Almonds have one of the highest levels of lean protein among all nuts. In addition to providing manganese and magnesium, almonds contribute a significant amount of vitamin E, an antioxidant that reduces oxygen free radicals, and oxidative stress, and protects against vascular damage and injury. They also contain unsaturated fats and fiber which help to reduce LDL (bad) cholesterol, blood pressure, blood glucose levels, and body weight.

CASHEWS: Cashews provide significant amounts of manganese, magnesium, and unsaturated fats, which helps reduce blood pressure, lowers LDL (bad) cholesterol, and therefore decreases the risk of cardiovascular diseases. Cashews are also rich in carotenoids and polyphenols, antioxidants that reduce oxygen free radicals, oxidative stress, and inflammation, which prevents vascular damage and injury.

PISTACHIOS: Pistachios are lower-calorie nuts that provide an excellent source of phosphorous and vitamins B1 and B6, which have significant antioxidant and anti-inflammatory properties, and therefore protect against vascular damage and injury. They also contain unsaturated fats and fiber which help to reduce LDL (bad) cholesterol, blood pressure, blood glucose levels, and body weight.

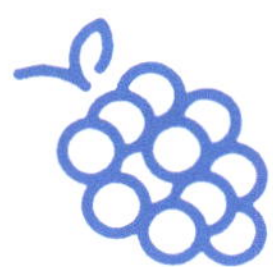

DRIED FRUITS – NO ADDED SUGAR

Dried fruits are portable and healthy snacks that can provide essential nutrients between meals. Different dried fruits contain varying levels of fiber, vitamins A, C, and E, potassium, magnesium, and antioxidants. Dried fruits contain more sugar than similar-sized pieces of fresh fruit because they are dehydrated and have less water. Moderate your consumption of dried fruit snacks because an excessive intake of natural sugars can elevate your blood glucose levels.

When buying dried fruit, select options that have no added sugar. Check the ingredients label on the package under "Carbohydrates" to ensure there is no added sugar.

RAISINS: This popular snack is an excellent source of fiber which lowers your LDL (bad) cholesterol, blood pressure, blood glucose, and body weight. Raisins are also a good source of potassium which lowers your risk of cardiovascular diseases by reducing blood pressure.

DRIED APRICOTS: Dried apricots are a high-fiber snack that helps reduce LDL (bad) cholesterol, blood pressure, blood glucose, and body weight. Apricots also contain flavonoids and vitamins A, C, and E, potent antioxidants that reduce oxygen free radicals, oxidative stress, and inflammation, which prevents vascular damage and injury.

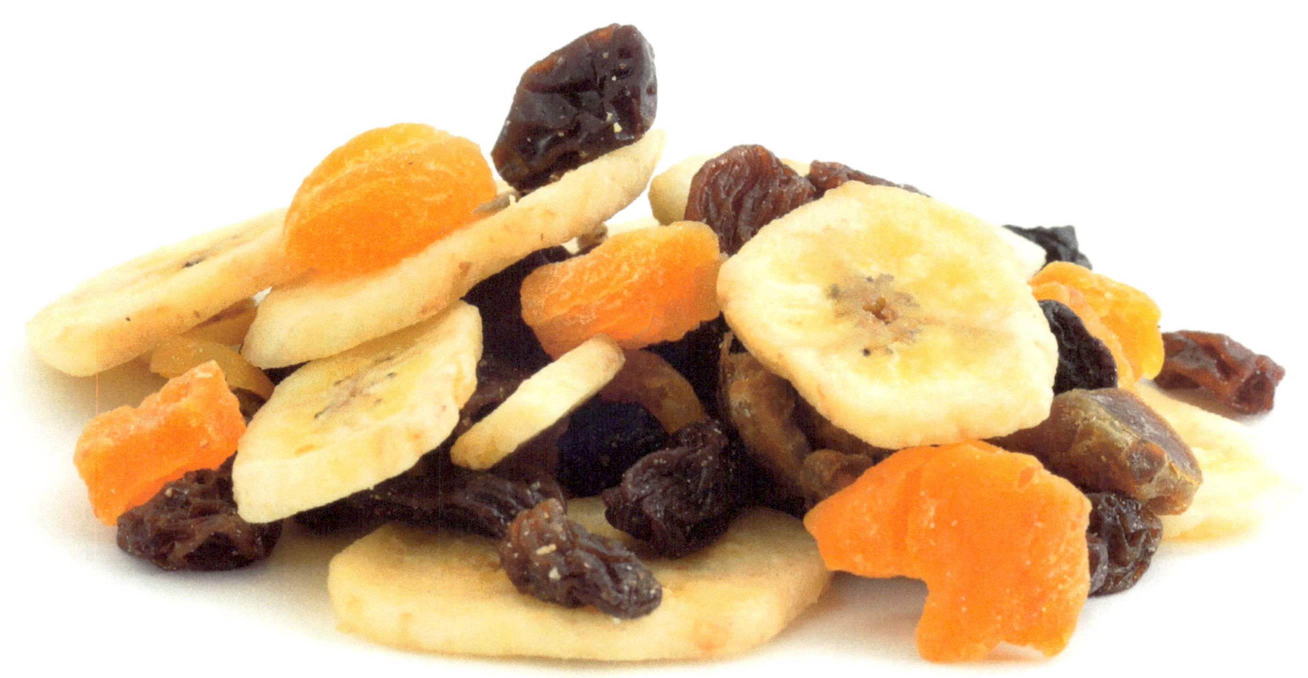

DRIED MANGOES: Mangoes are a great source of magnesium, potassium, and fiber, and therefore help lower blood pressure, LDL (bad) cholesterol, blood glucose, and body weight. Mangoes also contain vitamin C, a powerful antioxidant that reduces oxygen free radicals, oxidative stress, and vascular damage and injury.

Healthier Food Options

Many of the foods and beverages we consume are extremely unhealthy and increase the risk of cardiovascular diseases significantly. Therefore, as part of your Health Empowerment strategy, many common foods should be slowly reduced and eventually eliminated completely from your diet.

As you adopt a heart-healthy eating plan, you should *permanently replace* the following foods with healthier options, as noted.

ALL ADDED SALT, INCLUDING HIMALAYAN AND SEA SALT: All added sodium, no matter its source, significantly elevates blood pressure, which increases the risk of cardiovascular diseases. To flavor foods, replace salt with salt-free garlic and onion powder. Heart-healthy food has sufficient natural sodium for metabolism and should not be seasoned with salt.

ALL PROCESSED SUGAR, INCLUDING PROCESSED HONEY: All added sugar significantly elevates blood glucose, which increases the risk of diabetes, obesity, and cardiovascular diseases. Replace processed sugar with fresh fruits or unsweetened, unflavored, non-diary almond or oat-based milk to add a naturally sweet flavor to food and beverages. Heart-healthy food has sufficient natural sugars for metabolism.

ARTIFICIAL SWEETENERS: Research studies have revealed that artificial sweeteners (especially aspartame, acesulfame potassium, and sucralose) can elevate blood glucose and cause excessive weight gain with long-term use. In addition, some scientific organizations have expressed concern about a possible link between artificial sweeteners and certain cancers in humans. Replace these potentially harmful sweeteners with fresh fruits or unsweetened, unflavored, non-diary almond or oat-based milk to add a naturally sweet flavor to food and beverages.

SODA/SOFT DRINKS: The highly concentrated sugar content in soda significantly elevates blood glucose, which increases the risk of diabetes, obesity, and cardiovascular diseases. Replace soda with water or sugar-free, salt-free, no artificial sweetener, zero-calorie, flavored, or unflavored seltzer water.

PROCESSED JUICE, ENERGY DRINKS, AND STORE-PURCHASED FRUIT JUICES, INCLUDING ORANGE, APPLE, AND CRANBERRY: The highly concentrated sugar content in processed, store-purchased fruit juices significantly elevates blood glucose which increases the risk of diabetes, obesity, and cardiovascular diseases. Replace processed, store-purchased fruit juices with water or sugar-free, no artificial sweetener, zero-calorie iced tea.

NUTRIFACT:

Homemade freshly squeezed juices or smoothies with no added sugar or honey are healthier options than processed, store-purchased fruit juices, but fresh fruits and vegetables are healthiest when eaten whole because juicing and blending remove the fiber in the skin and pulp.

ALL DAIRY (COW'S) MILK/YOGURT, INCLUDING LACTAID, SKIM, 1 PERCENT, AND 2 PERCENT: All dairy milk contains excessive cholesterol and sugar, which significantly elevates blood cholesterol and blood glucose and increases the risk of dyslipidemia, diabetes, obesity, and cardiovascular diseases. Replace dairy milk/yogurt with unsweetened, unflavored, non-diary almond or oat-based milk/yogurt.

FLAVORED COFFEE CONTAINING SUGAR OR DAIRY MILK: Coffee beans contain naturally powerful antioxidants, including polyphenols, flavonoids, and chlorogenic acid, that reduce vascular inflammation, damage and injury, and the risk of cardiovascular diseases. Adding sugar, artificial sweeteners or dairy milk/creamer eliminates these benefits and makes your coffee unhealthy. Drink your coffee black/natural and sugar/sweetener-free, or with unsweetened, unflavored, non-dairy almond or oat-based milk only.

ALCOHOL BEVERAGES: Consuming limited alcohol (1-2 drinks) with family and friends during social and entertainment events like birthday and holiday celebrations can be safe. However, given the significant personal and public health risks (dependence, binge drinking, cardiovascular disease, liver disease, cognitive decline, driving while intoxicated) daily/frequent alcohol consumption, including wine, is not a recommended part of a heart-healthy nutrition plan.

PROCESSED/ULTRA-PROCESSED FOODS: Research studies have repeatedly demonstrated that foods manufactured with excessively added salt, sugar, saturated and trans fats, artificial flavors and colors, and preservatives, designed to improve shelf life, visual appeal, and taste, significantly increase the risk of hypertension, diabetes, dyslipidemia, obesity, atherosclerosis, and death from cardiovascular disease. Examples of processed/ultra-processed foods include potato chips, ice cream, cookies, donuts, processed meats (bacon, hot dogs, sausages), and frozen pizzas. Eliminate and replace these unhealthy foods with the natural and fresh foods on your Heart Food: Health Empowerment Shopping List.

CONDIMENTS: Many popular condiments, including ketchup, certain mustards, mayonnaise, hot sauces, butter, margarine, and salad dressings, are also processed/ultra-processed and manufactured with excessively added salt, sugar, saturated and trans fats, artificial flavors and colors, and preservatives making them extremely unhealthy. To ensure everything you eat promotes wellness only season and flavor your food with a variety of the heart-healthy condiments on your Heart Food: Health Empowerment Heart Shopping List and use homemade extra-virgin olive oil and vinegar salad dressing.

NUTRIFACT:

Unprocessed mustard made from natural mustard seeds, with no added salt, sugar, or honey, is heart-healthy when used in moderation. Mustard seeds are an excellent source of magnesium, manganese, phosphorus, copper, and vitamin B1, and they also contain essential omega-3 fatty acids, which are heart-healthy polyunsaturated fats.

GRADUAL PACE FOR ELIMINATING UNHEALTHY FOODS

Eliminating unhealthy foods can be challenging, to ensure a permanent transition to healthier options use this gradual pace strategy to permanently replace these food items as part of your Health Empowerment nutrition plan:

Select one day of the week to eliminate one unhealthy food from your diet for the first week, then introduce an additional day every week while never eating the unhealthy food on the days you already started. Start on the most convenient day for you and your family based on your schedule.

Example:

WEEK ONE: Eliminate one unhealthy food (for example seasoning with added salt) on Monday, and replace it with a healthier option (for example salt-free garlic or onion powder)

WEEK TWO: Never eat this unhealthy food on Mondays
Eliminate the unhealthy food on Tuesday

WEEK THREE: Never eat this unhealthy food on Mondays or Tuesdays
Eliminate the unhealthy food on Wednesday

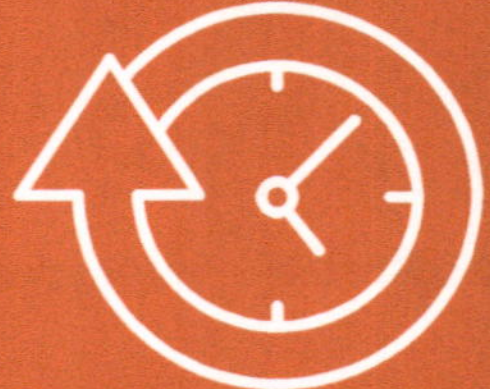

Continue this pattern for 7 weeks (approximately 1.5 months) until you have completely eliminated the selected unhealthy food, repeat this pattern for all the unhealthy foods in your diet one by one.

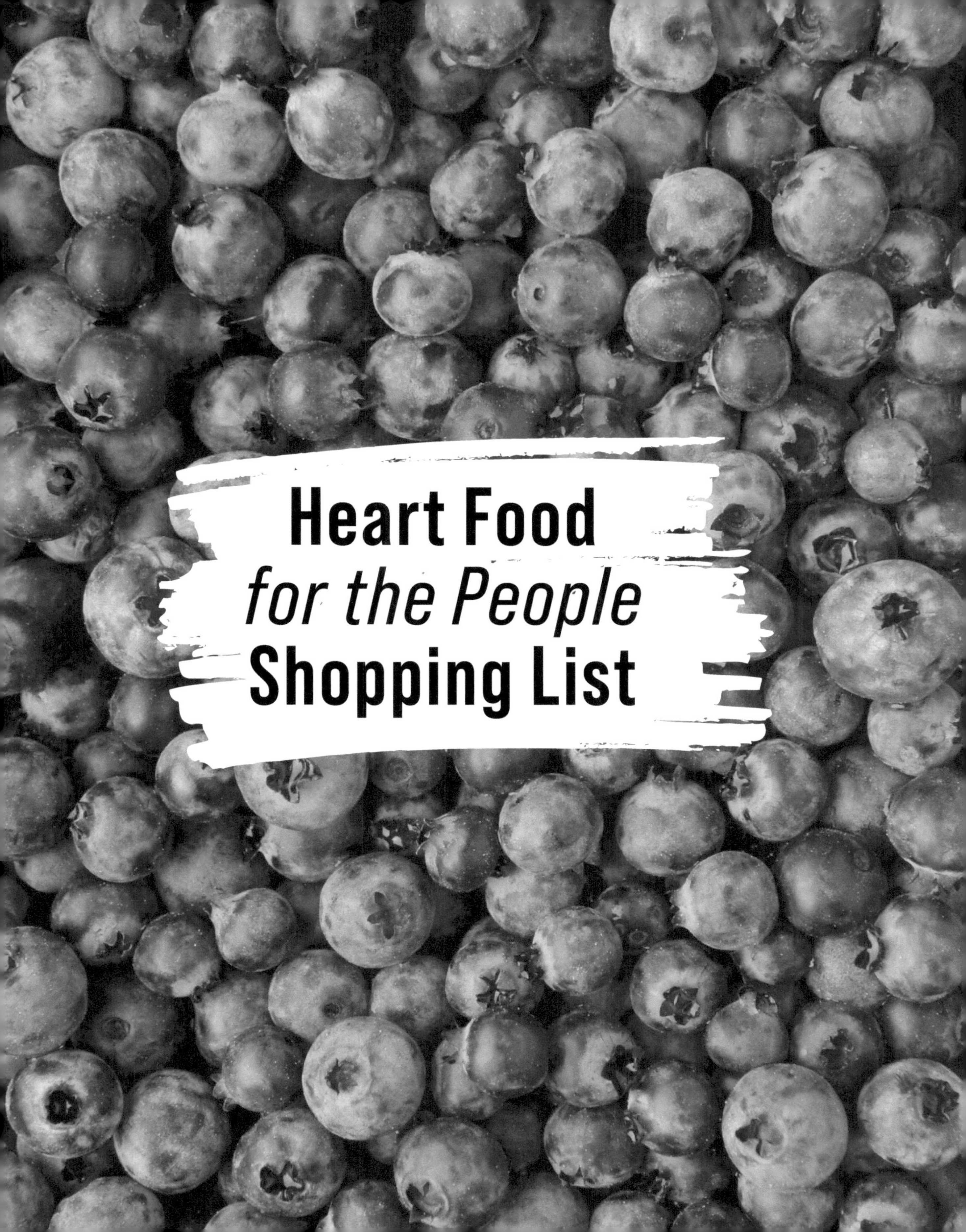
Heart Food
for the People
Shopping List

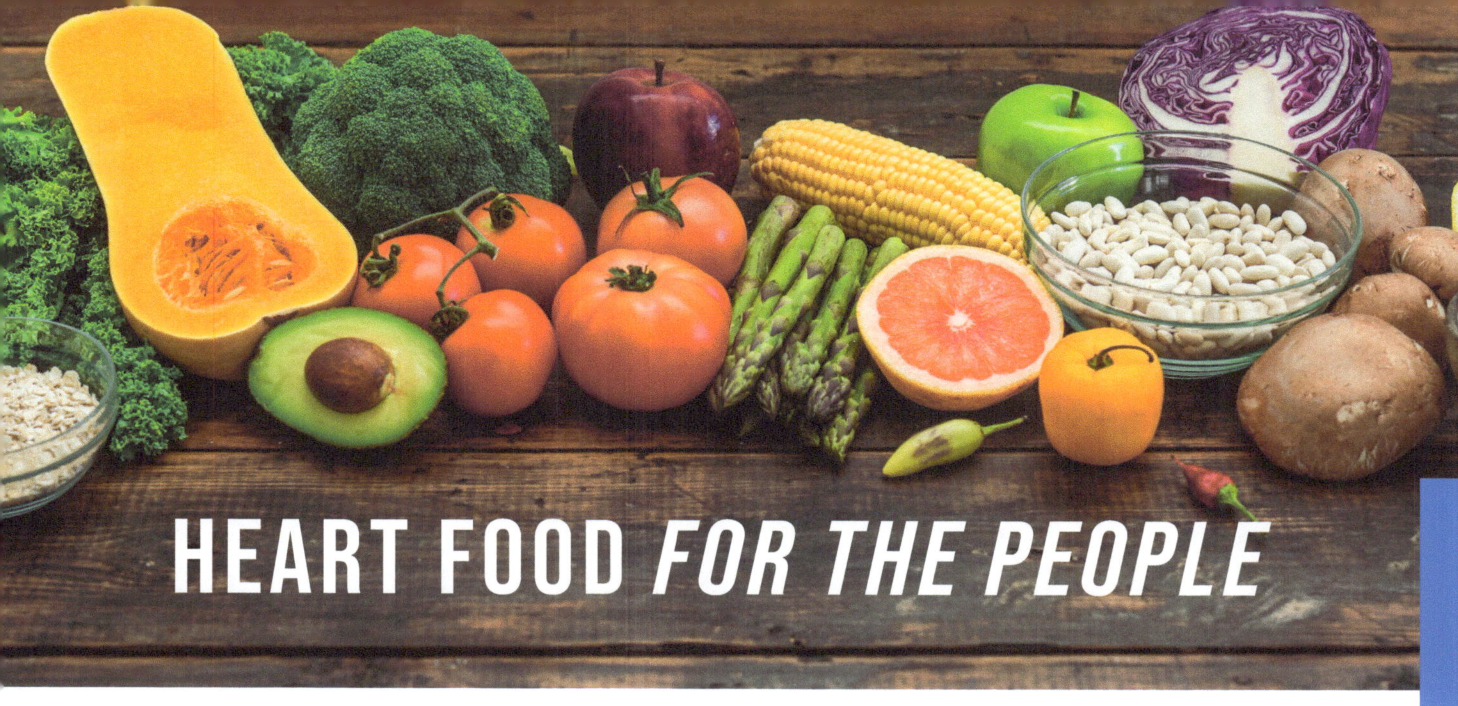

HEART FOOD *FOR THE PEOPLE*

Eating a heart-healthy diet starts with buying nutritious foods.

Heart-healthy nutrition involves a low-salt, lower-calorie, and primarily plant-based diet of fruits, vegetables, beans, nuts, oatmeal, whole grain wheat and bran cereals, non-dairy milk and yogurt, granola, complex carbohydrates, and extra-virgin olive oil, and lean meat proteins (primarily fish), and sugar-free beverages. This nutrition plan provides the essential balance of daily nutrients including enhanced lean protein, unsaturated fats, and fiber. It also ensures you eat the vitamins, minerals, and antioxidants necessary to sustain a heart-healthy diet. The evidence-based benefits of these foods have been well established and have been proven to promote wellness and prevent cardiovascular diseases.

Healthy foods can be hard to find and purchase in underserved communities because the realities of food deserts and food insecurity limit nutritious options. In addition, harmful and costly ultra-processed, junk, and fast foods are excessively promoted and marketed in underserved communities and are widely and easily available, which is an exploitative societal injustice and health inequity we must overcome with Health Empowerment. Using our resources to buy nutritious food available in the community is a vital part of that strategy.

We conducted detailed food accessibility and pricing surveys in over ten supermarkets and large grocery stores in multiple underserved communities and documented the heart-healthy foods we consistently found at affordable costs.

The following list reflects those options. While seemingly limited in variety and diversity, it represents the essential ingredients for a heart-healthy diet designed to facilitate a Health Empowerment strategy that will enable you to live longer and live better. Your unique shopping list may vary depending on your food allergies and the number of people in your household.

Heart Food:
Health Empowerment Shopping List

When available purchase store brands for reduced costs.

Read ingredients and labels carefully to ensure the following – salt-free, no added sodium, sugar-free, no added sugar, and no artificial sweeteners.

FRESH FRUIT

Purchase fresh fruits, no frozen or canned

- ☐ Raspberries
- ☐ Blueberries
- ☐ Strawberries
- ☐ Bananas
- ☐ Oranges
- ☐ Apples
- ☐ Red Grapes
- ☐ Limes

DRIED FRUIT

No added sugar

- ☐ Apricots
- ☐ Raisins
- ☐ Mangoes

VEGETABLES

Purchase fresh vegetables, no frozen or canned

- ☐ Baby Spinach
- ☐ Kale
- ☐ Red Onions
- ☐ Tomatoes
- ☐ Carrots
- ☐ Cucumbers
- ☐ Red Cabbage
- ☐ Broccoli
- ☐ Avocados
- ☐ Green, Yellow, and Red Bell Peppers
- ☐ Garlic

BEANS

Purchase canned, no added salt

Always drain and rinse beans with cold water before eating

- ☐ Kidney Beans
- ☐ Black Beans
- ☐ Chickpeas

OATS AND WHOLE GRAIN WHEAT AND BRAN CEREALS

No added sugar, unflavored

- ☐ Traditional Old-Fashioned Oatmeal
- ☐ Whole Grain Shredded Wheat Cereal
- ☐ Bran High-Fiber Cereal
- ☐ Classic Granola (whole grain rolled oats)

COMPLEX CARBOHYDRATES

- ☐ Brown Rice
- ☐ Sweet Potatoes (no frozen or canned)

LEAN (LOW-FAT) MEAT PROTEIN

- ☐ Salmon
- ☐ Cod loin filet
- ☐ Tilapia
- ☐ Skinless, boneless chicken breast

YOGURT

- ☐ Non-Dairy Yogurt, Almond or Oat-Based — Unsweetened, Unflavored

NUTS

Raw, no added salt or sugar/honey

- ☐ Almonds
- ☐ Pistachios
- ☐ Walnuts
- ☐ Cashews

- ☐ Extra-Virgin Olive Oil
- ☐ Red Wine Vinegar
- ☐ Apple Cider Vinegar
- ☐ Garlic Powder (salt-free)
- ☐ Onion Powder (salt-free)
- ☐ Black Pepper
- ☐ Oregano
- ☐ Paprika
- ☐ Cumin
- ☐ Cayenne Pepper

- ☐ Water
- ☐ Non-dairy Milk — Almond or Oat-based, Unsweetened, Unflavored
- ☐ Seltzer Water — Sugar-Free, Salt-Free, no Artificial Sweetener, Zero-Calorie, Flavored, or Unflavored
- ☐ Iced Tea — Sugar-Free, no Artificial Sweetener, Zero-Calorie

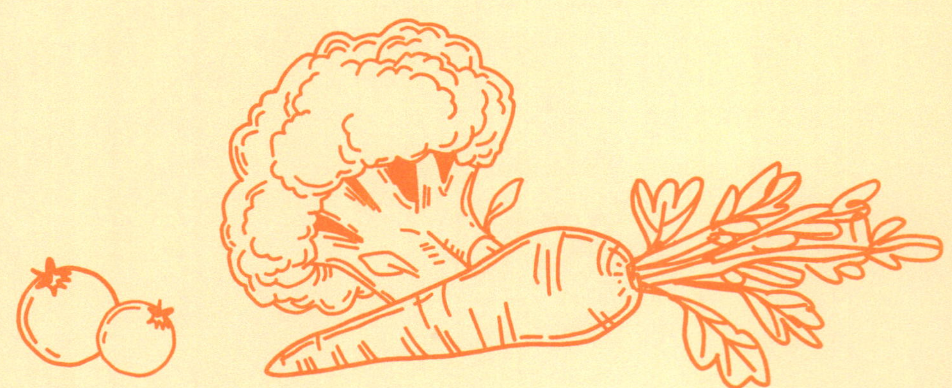

If a food category is not on the Heart Food: Health Empowerment Shopping List it is not heart-healthy and ideally should not be a part of your Health Empowerment nutrition plan

examples: beef, pork, eggs, cheese, shellfish (shrimp, clams, scallops, crab, lobster)

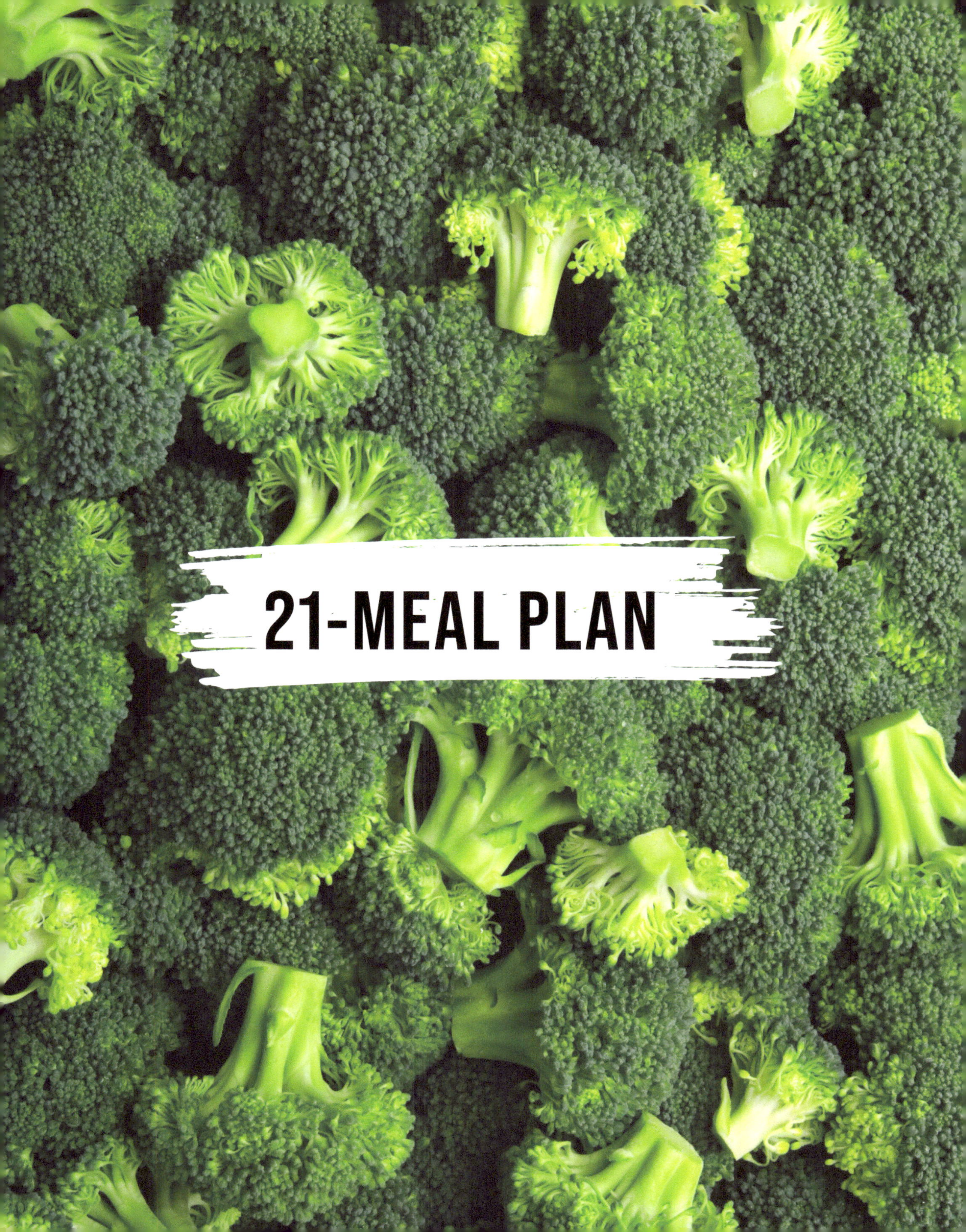

21-MEAL PLAN

MEAL PLAN

The foods from the Heart Food: Health Empowerment Shopping List represent the most important element of a Health Empowerment strategy and contain the nutrients we need to promote wellness. When eaten daily, these foods have the potential to prevent cardiovascular diseases. Nutritious food is ultimately the greatest resource underserved communities have to promote wellness, independent of the healthcare system.

Following, you will find 21 simple, easy-to-prepare, heart-healthy meals for breakfast, lunch, and dinner for one full week. The meals follow a consistent pattern, using the same category of food types for each meal. Once you are comfortable with the main ingredients, you will be able to create your own unique versions of the Health Empowerment heart-healthy nutrition plan. In addition, two heart-healthy snacks are included each day, to ensure everything you eat will make you live longer and live better.

MEAL BASICS

The basic food groups for every meal and snack in the plan include:

> **BREAKFAST** – a 12-ounce bowl of cooked traditional old-fashioned oatmeal with unsweetened, unflavored, non-dairy milk (almond or oat-based); or a 12-ounce bowl of cold whole grain shredded wheat or bran high-fiber cereal

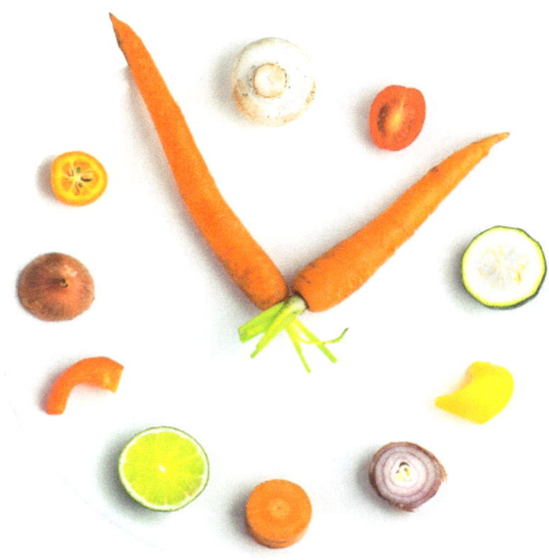

with unsweetened, unflavored, non-dairy milk (almond or oat-based); or a 12-ounce bowl of unsweetened, unflavored, non-dairy yogurt (almond or oat-based) with granola – each option always with three different fresh fruits added to the oatmeal, cereal or yogurt

LUNCH – a cold salad with a leafy green base (spinach or kale), a bean protein source (canned, uncooked, no added salt, kidney beans, black beans, or chickpeas), four additional different vegetables, and homemade extra-virgin olive oil and vinegar salad dressing with a variety of added condiments

DINNER – a half plate of vegetables (one or more, cold or cooked), a quarter plate of complex carbohydrates (sweet potatoes or brown rice), a quarter plate of lean meat protein (sauteed or baked fish or skinless chicken breast)

HEART-HEALTHY SNACKS – mid-morning / mid-afternoon snack – raw nuts with no added salt or sugar/honey, or dried fruits with no added sugar; after-dinner snack – two fresh fruits ½ cup each

In addition to the above, eat 1 – 2 garlic cloves daily (raw – chopped or minced). Allicin, the powerful antioxidant in garlic, reduces LDL (bad) cholesterol, blood glucose, and blood pressure, and it enhances the function of other natural antioxidants in the body and therefore has an amplifying effect to prevent cardiovascular diseases. The Health Empowerment meal plans incorporate this recommendation.

These meals may represent a significant transition from the way you are currently eating. Since it may be challenging logistically, financially, and psychologically to change your diet all at once, we recommend you start at your own pace. While we suggest traditional meals for breakfast, lunch, and dinner, you can switch the time of day you prefer to eat each one. Use one of the following strategies based on your unique reality to start your Health Empowerment nutrition plan.

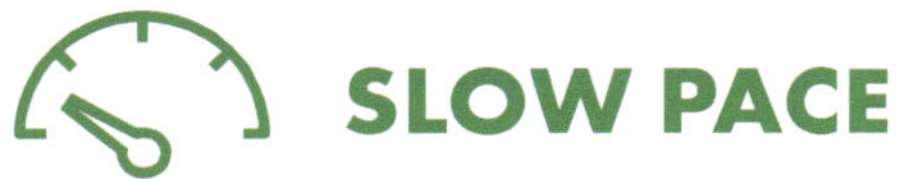

SLOW PACE

New dietary strategies take time to develop. To ensure success, consider this slow pace transition to gradually incorporate all 21 meals into your nutrition plan:

Select one single meal from the meal plan to eat the first week, and add a new meal weekly while always continuing the meals you already started. Start with one meal on the most convenient day for you and your family.

Example:

WEEK ONE: Start Day 1 Breakfast on Saturday

WEEK TWO: Continue Day 1 Breakfast every Saturday
Start Day 2 Breakfast on Sunday

WEEK THREE: Continue Day 1 Breakfast every Saturday
Continue Day 2 Breakfast every Sunday
Start Day 3 Breakfast on Monday

Continue this pattern for 21 weeks (approximately 5 months) until you have incorporated every meal into your diet.

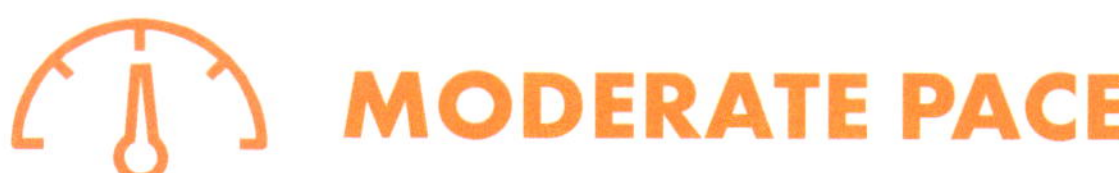

New dietary strategies take time to develop. To ensure success, consider this moderate pace transition to gradually incorporate all 21 meals into your nutrition plan:

Select two meals from the meal plan to eat the first week, and add two new meals weekly while always continuing the meals you already started. Start with two meals on the most convenient day for you and your family.

Example:

WEEK ONE:
Start Day 1 Breakfast on Monday
Start Day 1 Dinner on Monday

WEEK TWO:
Continue Day 1 Breakfast every Monday
Continue Day 1 Dinner every Monday
Start Day 2 Breakfast on Tuesday
Start Day 2 Dinner on Tuesday

WEEK THREE:
Continue Day 1 Breakfast every Monday
Continue Day 1 Dinner every Monday
Continue Day 2 Breakfast every Tuesday
Continue Day 2 Dinner every Tuesday
Start Day 3 Breakfast on Wednesday
Start Day 3 Dinner on Wednesday

Continue this pattern for 11 weeks (approximately 2.5 months) until you have incorporated every meal into your diet

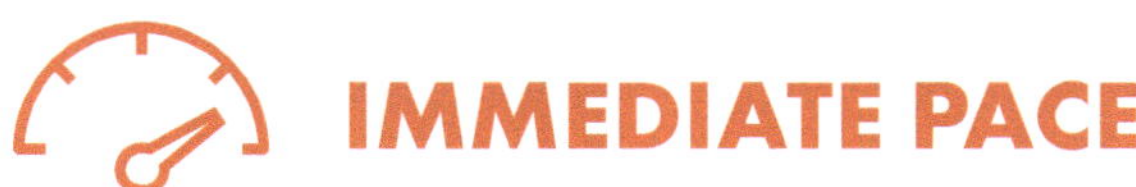

If you have the resources and time, you can choose to eat all your meals from the 21-meal plan immediately. Incorporating all 21 meals on the plan at once will require a concerted commitment and effort, especially if the meal plan represents a significant transition from your previous diet. However, with this strategy, you will experience a rapid improvement in your health and energy.

The Health Empowerment strategy also ensures that the food you eat is based on the essential balance of daily nutrients necessary to sustain a heart-healthy diet. Detailed explanations of why each food is heart-healthy are included with every meal and snack to confirm you understand and feel confident that everything you eat promotes wellness.

In addition, estimates of food content regarding calories and macronutrients are provided for every meal and snack, and a daily total is also included. These can be compared to recommended daily allowances for reference.

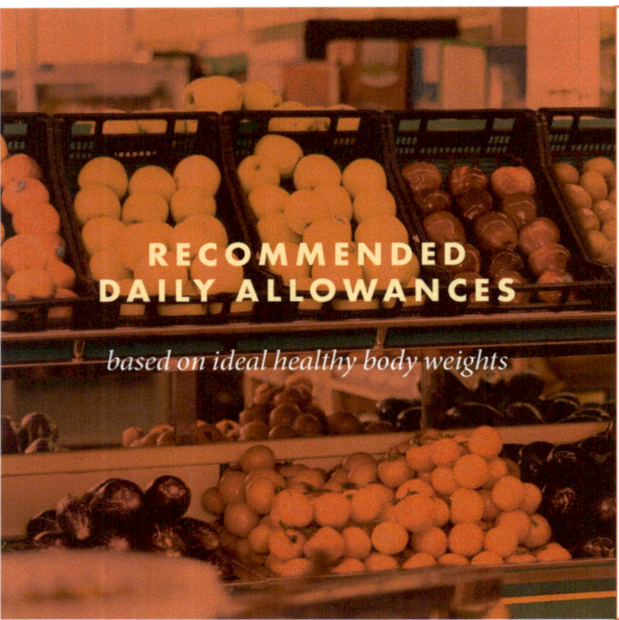

TOTAL DAILY CALORIES: 2000 – 2500 calories

TOTAL DAILY LEAN (LOW-FAT) PROTEIN: 55 – 60 grams (gm)

TOTAL DAILY COMPLEX CARBOHYDRATES: 225 – 325 grams (gm)

TOTAL DAILY UNSATURATED (MONO AND POLYUNSATURATED) FATS: 45 – 60 grams (gm)

TOTAL DAILY FIBER: 25 – 30 grams (gm)

The Health Empowerment nutrition plan incorporates evidenced-based strategies that emphasize a low-salt, lower-calorie, and primarily plant-based diet of fruits, vegetables, beans, nuts, oatmeal, whole grain wheat and bran cereals, non-dairy milk and yogurt, granola, complex carbohydrates, and extra-virgin olive oil, and lean meat proteins (primarily fish), and sugar-free beverages. This nutrition plan provides the essential balance of daily nutrients including enhanced lean protein, unsaturated fats and fiber, and vitamins, minerals, and antioxidants necessary to sustain a heart-healthy diet, promote wellness, and significantly reduce the risk of cardiovascular diseases.

The Health Empowerment meal plans should be followed as closely as possible to maximize health benefits.

Each dinner in the 21-meal plan follows the perfect plate model, a meal-planning strategy that provides the right balance of nutrients and calories. This includes half a plate of vegetables (one or more, cold or cooked), a quarter plate of complex carbohydrates (sweet potatoes, brown rice), and a quarter plate of lean meat protein (fish, skinless chicken breast).

In addition to food, you should drink at least eight to ten cups (½ gallon, 2 liters) of water a day for optimal health, and for variety only substitute water with the sugar-free, unsweetened, and zero-calorie beverages

on the Heart Food: Health Empowerment Shopping List (seltzer water, iced tea).

NUTRIFACT:

When possible, add freshly squeezed lime juice (½ lime) to your drinking water for added vitamin C which is a powerful antioxidant that reduces oxygen free radicals, oxidative stress, and inflammation, which prevents vascular damage and injury. In addition, fresh lime juice also provides potassium and magnesium, essential minerals that maintain proper water and electrolyte balance and therefore help reduce blood pressure and prevent hypertension.

The **Meal/Snack Benefits** described below each meal and snack ensure you understand in detail how the foods you eat provide a nutrient balance that is designed to promote wellness and prevent cardiovascular diseases.

The **Meal/Snack and Daily Total Calculations** are estimates of caloric and macronutrient content based on reported food properties meant to serve as a guide to ensure you feel confident that the Health Empowerment nutrition plan provides the optimal balance of energy and macronutrients relative to recommended daily allowances. They are not precise, scientifically conducted measurements.

BREAKFAST

OATMEAL WITH FRESH FRUIT

- 12-ounce bowl of traditional old-fashioned oatmeal cooked with 1½ cups unsweetened, unflavored non-dairy milk (almond or oat-based)
- ½ cup raspberries
- ½ banana
- ½ cup blueberries

no added sugar or honey

Meal Benefits

OATMEAL – contains a high concentration of the soluble fiber beta-glucan, which reduces LDL (bad) cholesterol, blood glucose, blood pressure, and body weight and therefore helps prevent atherosclerosis, diabetes, hypertension, and obesity; beta-glucan also promotes healthy gut bacteria and intestinal health which reduces systemic inflammation that contributes to vascular damage and injury; also contributes vitamin B1, manganese, and phytonutrients, potent antioxidants that reduce oxygen free radicals, oxidative stress, and inflammation, which prevents vascular damage and injury.

NON-DAIRY MILK (ALMOND OR OAT-BASED) – contains no cholesterol, and lower total calories and sugar than dairy milk, reducing the risk of atherosclerosis and diabetes; also contributes lean protein and calcium, two nutrients that help sustain healthy vascular function, regulate normal blood pressure, and prevent hypertension.

RASPBERRIES – contain anthocyanins, antioxidants that reduce oxygen free radicals, oxidative stress, and inflammation, which prevents vascular damage and injury; also provide a high concentration of soluble fiber, potassium, and manganese which reduces LDL (bad) cholesterol, blood glucose, body weight, and blood pressure and therefore helps prevent atherosclerosis, diabetes, obesity, and hypertension.

BANANA – contains vitamin C, an antioxidant that reduces oxygen free radicals, oxidative stress, and inflammation, which prevents vascular damage and injury; also contains a high concentration of potassium and fiber, which helps prevent hypertension, atherosclerosis, diabetes, and obesity by reducing blood pressure, LDL (bad) cholesterol, blood glucose, and body weight.

BLUEBERRIES – contain the highest concentration of the antioxidants anthocyanins among all fresh fruits, reducing oxygen free radicals, oxidative stress, and inflammation, which prevents vascular damage and injury; also contain a high concentration of vitamin C and soluble fiber, which reduces blood pressure, LDL (bad) cholesterol, blood glucose, and body weight and therefore helps prevent hypertension, atherosclerosis, diabetes, and obesity.

Breakfast Calculations

Meal Total	Calories	Lean Protein	Complex Carbohydrates	Unsaturated Fat	Fiber
	554	17 gm	110 gm	9 gm	18 gm

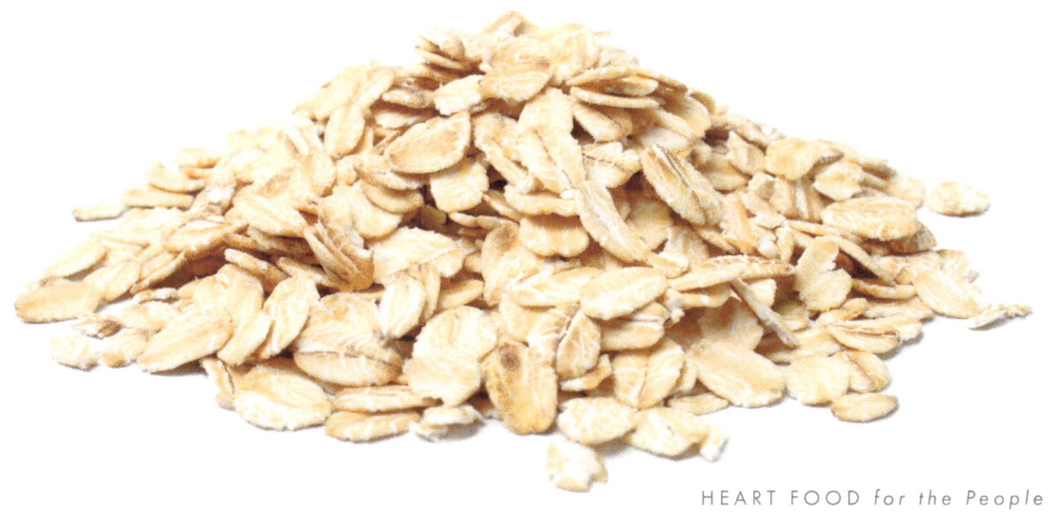

LUNCH

VEGETABLE SALAD WITH KIDNEY BEANS

- 2 cups baby spinach
- 1 cup kidney beans *(drain and rinse with cold water before eating)*
- ½ cucumber
- ½ cup tomatoes
- ½ cup carrots
- ½ red onion, sliced

Olive oil vinaigrette – mix and add as salad dressing

- 2 tablespoons extra-virgin olive oil
- 1 tablespoon red wine vinegar
- 1 teaspoon black pepper

Meal Benefits

SPINACH – contains phytonutrients and vitamin C, potent antioxidants that reduce oxygen free radicals, oxidative stress, and inflammation, which prevents vascular damage and injury; also contributes vitamin D, calcium, and fiber, which reduces blood pressure, LDL (bad) cholesterol, blood glucose, and body weight and therefore helps prevent hypertension, atherosclerosis, diabetes, and obesity.

KIDNEY BEANS — contain lean protein, iron, and soluble fiber, which sustains healthy vascular function, prevents anemia, reduces blood pressure, LDL (bad) cholesterol, blood glucose, and body weight, and therefore helps prevent hypertension, atherosclerosis, diabetes, and obesity.

CUCUMBER UNPEELED (PEELING REDUCES THE AMOUNT OF FIBER, VITAMINS, AND MINERALS) – contains vitamin C, a strong antioxidant that reduces oxygen free radicals, oxidative stress, and inflammation, which prevents vascular damage and injury; provides magnesium and potassium, essential minerals that help maintain proper water and electrolyte balance to sustain normal blood pressure and prevent hypertension; also provides fiber, which reduces LDL (bad) cholesterol, blood glucose, and body weight, and therefore helps prevent atherosclerosis, diabetes, and obesity.

TOMATOES – contain lycopene and vitamins B, C, and E, powerful antioxidants that reduce oxygen free radicals, oxidative stress, and inflammation, which prevents vascular damage and injury; also contain a high concentration of potassium, which lowers blood pressure to prevent hypertension.

CARROTS – contain vitamins A and C, and beta-carotene, strong antioxidants that reduce oxygen free radicals, oxidative stress, and inflammation, which prevents vascular damage and injury; also contribute fiber, which reduces LDL (bad) cholesterol, blood glucose, blood pressure, and body weight and therefore helps prevent atherosclerosis, diabetes, hypertension, and obesity.

RED ONIONS – contain the powerful antioxidants quercetin and vitamin C that reduce oxygen free radicals, oxidative stress, and inflammation, which prevents vascular damage and injury; also contribute calcium and fiber, which reduces blood pressure, LDL (bad) cholesterol, blood glucose, and body weight and therefore helps prevent hypertension, atherosclerosis, diabetes, and obesity.

OLIVE OIL – contains a high concentration of oleocanthal and vitamin E, powerful antioxidants that reduce oxygen free radicals, oxidative stress, and inflammation, which prevents vascular damage and injury; also provides a high concentration of monounsaturated fats, which lowers LDL (bad) cholesterol, increases HDL (good) cholesterol and therefore helps prevent atherosclerosis.

RED WINE VINEGAR – contains polyphenols, powerful antioxidants that reduce oxygen free radicals, oxidative stress, and inflammation, which prevents vascular damage and injury; also contains acetic acid which lowers LDL (bad) cholesterol, blood pressure, blood glucose levels, and body weight and therefore helps prevent atherosclerosis, hypertension, diabetes, and obesity.

BLACK PEPPER –contains the powerful antioxidant piperine that reduces oxygen free radicals, oxidative stress, and inflammation, which prevents vascular damage and injury; also contains potassium, calcium, and magnesium, essential minerals that lower blood pressure and LDL (bad) cholesterol levels and therefore help prevent hypertension and atherosclerosis.

Lunch Calculations

Meal Total	Calories	Lean Protein	Complex Carbohydrates	Unsaturated Fat	Fiber
	422	10 gm	36 gm	28 gm	12 gm

HEART-HEALTHY SNACK

(could be divided between mid-morning and mid-afternoon)

- ½ cup whole almonds (*raw, no added salt or sugar/honey*)

Snack Benefits

ALMONDS – contain high levels of lean protein, unsaturated fats, and fiber, which sustains healthy vascular function, reduces LDL (bad) cholesterol, blood glucose, and body weight, and therefore helps prevent hypertension, atherosclerosis, diabetes, and obesity; also contribute significant amounts of manganese and magnesium, essential minerals which also helps lower blood pressure and LDL (bad) cholesterol.

Snack Calculations

Snack Total	Calories	Lean Protein	Complex Carbohydrates	Unsaturated Fat	Fiber
	138	5 gm	0 gm	12 gm	3 gm

DINNER

SAUTEED SALMON AND STEAMED GARLIC BROCCOLI WITH BROWN RICE

- 6 ounces of sauteed salmon
- 1 tablespoon extra-virgin olive oil (use to sauté salmon)
- half a plate steamed broccoli mixed with 1 garlic clove, minced
- 1 cup brown rice
- 1 tablespoon fresh lime juice (add to salmon or broccoli)

Season dinner meals with your choice and preference from the powdered condiments on the shopping list – salt-free garlic and onion powder are especially healthy options. Gradually eliminate seasoning food with salt as previously described in the Healthier Food Options section.

Meal Benefits

SALMON – contains high concentrations of vitamins B6 and B12, which helps maintain healthy red blood cells, prevents anemia, and therefore reduces the risk of vascular damage and injury; also provides a high concentration of polyunsaturated fats called omega-3 fatty acids, which lowers LDL (bad) cholesterol, increases HDL (good) cholesterol and therefore helps prevent atherosclerosis.

BROCCOLI – contains flavonoids, carotenoids including lutein and beta-carotene, and vitamin C, which are powerful antioxidants that reduce oxygen free radicals, oxidative stress, and inflammation, which prevents vascular damage and injury; also contains a high concentration of soluble fiber, which reduces LDL (bad) cholesterol, blood glucose, blood pressure, and body weight, and therefore helps prevent atherosclerosis, diabetes, hypertension, and obesity.

GARLIC – contains allicin, a powerful antioxidant that reduces oxygen free radicals, oxidative stress, and inflammation, which prevents vascular damage and injury; also contains vitamin C and fiber, which reduces blood pressure, LDL (bad) cholesterol, blood glucose, and body weight and therefore helps prevent hypertension, atherosclerosis, diabetes, and obesity.

BROWN RICE (WHOLE GRAIN, MOST OF THE VITAMINS AND MINERALS ARE IN THE TWO OUTER LAYERS OF RICE) – a complex carbohydrate low on the glycemic index (an index that measures how much a food increases your blood sugar levels) and rich in lean protein, calcium, iron, magnesium, and soluble fiber, which sustains healthy vascular function and reduces LDL (bad) cholesterol, blood glucose, and body weight, and therefore helps prevent hypertension, atherosclerosis, diabetes, and obesity; also contains flavonoid antioxidants that reduce oxygen free radicals, oxidative stress, and inflammation, which prevents vascular damage and injury.

LIME JUICE, FRESH – contains a high concentration of vitamin C, which is a powerful antioxidant that reduces oxygen free radicals, oxidative stress, and inflammation, which prevents vascular damage and injury; also provides potassium and magnesium, essential minerals that maintain proper water and electrolyte balance and therefore help reduce blood pressure and prevent hypertension.

OLIVE OIL – contains a high concentration of oleocanthal and vitamin E, powerful antioxidants that reduce oxygen free radicals, oxidative stress, and inflammation, which prevents vascular damage and injury; also provides a high concentration of monounsaturated fats, which lowers LDL (bad) cholesterol, increases HDL (good) cholesterol and therefore helps prevent atherosclerosis.

Dinner Calculations

Meal Total	Calories	Lean Protein	Complex Carbohydrates	Unsaturated Fat	Fiber
	660	54 gm	41 gm	31 gm	3 gm

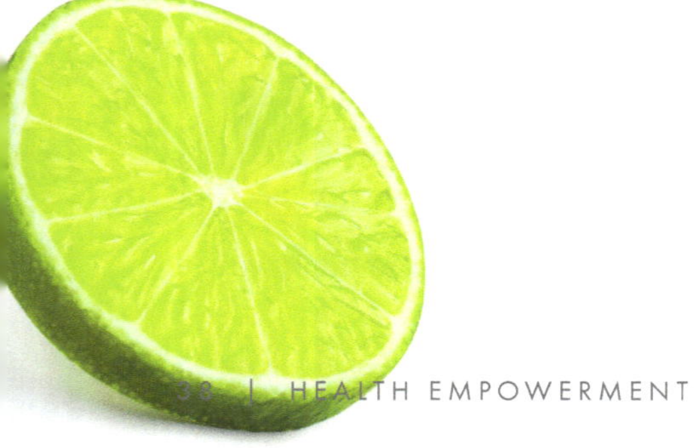

DAY 1

HEART-HEALTHY SNACK

(eat at least several hours before going to sleep)

- ½ cup red grapes
- ½ cup strawberries

Snack Benefits

RED GRAPES – contain a high concentration of potassium, which helps maintain proper water and electrolyte balance to sustain normal blood pressure and prevent hypertension; also contain resveratrol and vitamin C, strong antioxidants that reduce oxygen free radicals, oxidative stress, and inflammation, which prevents vascular damage and injury.

STRAWBERRIES – contain the antioxidants vitamin C, anthocyanins, and quercetin that reduce oxygen free radicals, oxidative stress, and inflammation, which prevents vascular damage and injury; also contribute soluble fiber, which reduces LDL (bad) cholesterol, blood glucose, blood pressure, and body weight and therefore helps prevent atherosclerosis, diabetes, hypertension, and obesity.

Snack Calculations

Snack Total	Calories	Lean Protein	Complex Carbohydrates	Unsaturated Fat	Fiber
	110	1 gm	27 gm	0 gm	4 gm

Daily Total Calculations

Daily Total	Calories	Lean Protein	Complex Carbohydrates	Unsaturated Fat	Fiber
	1884	87 gm	214 gm	80 gm	40 gm

BREAKFAST

WHOLE GRAIN SHREDDED WHEAT OR BRAN HIGH-FIBER CEREAL WITH FRESH FRUIT

- 12-ounce bowl of whole grain shredded wheat or bran high-fiber cereal
- 1½ cups unsweetened, unflavored non-dairy milk (almond or oat-based)
- ½ banana
- ½ cup blueberries
- ½ cup strawberries

no added sugar or honey

Meal Benefits

WHOLE GRAIN SHREDDED WHEAT OR BRAN HIGH-FIBER CEREAL – contains a high concentration of fiber, which reduces LDL (bad) cholesterol, blood glucose, blood pressure, and body weight and therefore helps prevent atherosclerosis, diabetes, hypertension, and obesity; fiber also promotes healthy gut bacteria and intestinal health which reduces systemic inflammation that contributes to vascular damage and injury; also an excellent source of phosphorous which has significant antioxidant properties that reduce oxygen free radicals, oxidative stress, and inflammation, helping to prevent atherosclerosis.

NON-DAIRY MILK (ALMOND OR OAT-BASED) – contains no cholesterol, and lower total calories and sugar than dairy milk, reducing the risk of atherosclerosis and diabetes; also contributes lean protein and calcium, two nutrients that help sustain healthy vascular function, regulate normal blood pressure, and prevent hypertension.

BANANA – contains vitamin C, an antioxidant that reduces oxygen free radicals, oxidative stress, and inflammation, which prevents vascular damage and injury; also contains a high concentration of potassium and fiber, which helps prevent hypertension, atherosclerosis, diabetes, and obesity by reducing blood pressure, LDL (bad) cholesterol, blood glucose, and body weight.

BLUEBERRIES – contain the highest concentration of the antioxidants anthocyanins among all fresh fruits, reducing oxygen free radicals, oxidative stress, and inflammation, which prevents vascular damage and injury; also contain a high concentration of vitamin C and soluble fiber, which reduces blood pressure, LDL (bad) cholesterol, blood glucose, and body

weight and therefore helps prevent hypertension, atherosclerosis, diabetes, and obesity.

STRAWBERRIES – contain the antioxidants vitamin C, anthocyanins, and quercetin that reduce oxygen free radicals, oxidative stress, and inflammation, which prevents vascular damage and injury; also contribute soluble fiber, which reduces LDL (bad) cholesterol, blood glucose, blood pressure, and body weight and therefore helps prevent atherosclerosis, diabetes, hypertension, and obesity.

Breakfast Calculations

Meal Total	Calories	Lean Protein	Complex Carbohydrates	Unsaturated Fat	Fiber
	569	18 gm	122 gm	6 gm	20 gm

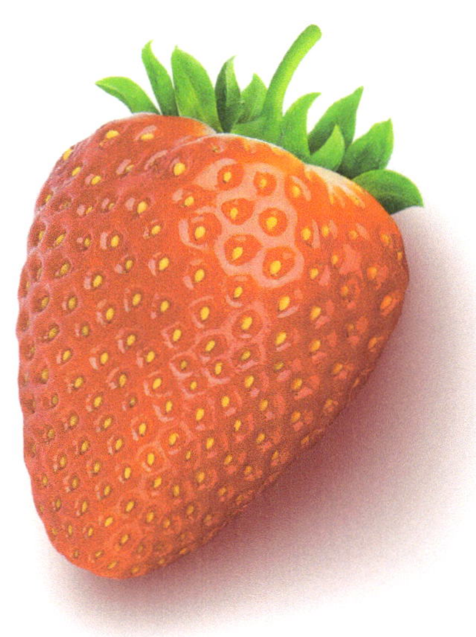

LUNCH

VEGETABLE SALAD WITH BLACK BEANS

- 2 cups kale
- 1 cup black beans (*drain and rinse with cold water before eating*)
- ½ cup uncooked broccoli
- ½ avocado
- ½ green bell pepper
- 1 garlic clove, chopped

Olive oil vinaigrette – mix and add as salad dressing

- 2 tablespoons extra-virgin olive oil
- 1 tablespoon apple wine vinegar
- 1 teaspoon oregano

Meal Benefits

KALE – contains vitamin C and phytonutrients, antioxidants that reduce oxygen free radicals, oxidative stress, and inflammation, which prevents vascular damage and injury; also contains vitamin D, calcium, and fiber, which reduces blood pressure, LDL (bad) cholesterol, blood glucose, and body weight and therefore helps prevent hypertension, atherosclerosis, diabetes, and obesity.

BLACK BEANS — contain lean protein, iron, and soluble fiber, which sustains healthy vascular function, prevents anemia, reduces blood pressure, LDL (bad) cholesterol, blood glucose, and body weight, and therefore helps prevent atherosclerosis, hypertension, diabetes, and obesity.

BROCCOLI – contains flavonoids, carotenoids including lutein and beta-carotene, and vitamin C, which are powerful antioxidants that reduce oxygen free radicals, oxidative stress, and inflammation, which prevents vascular damage and injury; also contains a high concentration of soluble fiber, which reduces LDL (bad) cholesterol, blood glucose, blood pressure, and body weight, and therefore helps prevent atherosclerosis, diabetes, hypertension, and obesity.

AVOCADO – contains healthy monounsaturated fats, which lowers LDL (bad) cholesterol, increases HDL (good) cholesterol, and therefore helps prevent atherosclerosis; contributes the antioxidants vitamins C and E, and copper that reduce oxygen free radicals, oxidative stress, and inflammation, which prevents vascular damage and injury; also provides manganese which reduces blood pressure and therefore helps prevent hypertension.

GREEN BELL PEPPER – contains high levels of the antioxidants vitamins C and B6 that reduce oxygen free radicals, oxidative stress, and inflammation, which prevents vascular damage and injury; also contributes potassium and soluble fiber, which reduces blood pressure, LDL (bad) cholesterol, blood glucose, and body weight and therefore helps prevent hypertension, atherosclerosis, diabetes, and obesity.

GARLIC – contains allicin, a powerful antioxidant that reduces oxygen free radicals, oxidative stress, and inflammation, which prevents vascular damage and injury; also contains vitamin C and fiber, which reduces blood pressure, LDL (bad) cholesterol, blood glucose, and body weight and therefore helps prevent hypertension, atherosclerosis, diabetes, and obesity.

OLIVE OIL – contains a high concentration of oleocanthal and vitamin E, powerful antioxidants that reduce oxygen free radicals, oxidative stress, and inflammation, which prevents vascular damage and injury; also provides a high concentration of monounsaturated fats, which lowers LDL (bad) cholesterol, increases HDL (good) cholesterol and therefore helps prevent atherosclerosis.

APPLE WINE VINEGAR – contains polyphenols, powerful antioxidants that reduce oxygen free radicals, oxidative stress, and inflammation, which prevents vascular damage and injury; also contains acetic acid which lowers LDL (bad) cholesterol, blood pressure, blood glucose levels, and body weight and therefore helps prevent atherosclerosis, hypertension, diabetes, and obesity.

OREGANO – contains a high concentration of polyphenol antioxidants, including carvacrol, that reduce oxygen free radicals, oxidative stress, and inflammation, which prevents vascular damage and injury; also provides high levels of calcium, which is essential to normal cardiac and vascular function and helps reduce blood pressure and therefore prevent hypertension.

Lunch Calculations

Meal Total	Calories	Lean Protein	Complex Carbohydrates	Unsaturated Fat	Fiber
	583	16 gm	47 gm	40 gm	22 gm

HEART-HEALTHY SNACK

(could be divided between mid-morning and mid-afternoon)

- ½ cup dried apricots (*no added sugar*)

Snack Benefits

DRIED APRICOTS – contain a high concentration of flavonoids and vitamins A, C, and E, potent antioxidants that reduce oxygen free radicals, oxidative stress, and inflammation, which prevents vascular damage and injury; also an excellent source of fiber which helps reduce blood pressure, LDL (bad) cholesterol, blood glucose, and body weight.

Snack Calculations

Snack Total	Calories	Lean Protein	Complex Carbohydrates	Unsaturated Fat	Fiber
	200	2 gm	48 gm	0 gm	4 gm

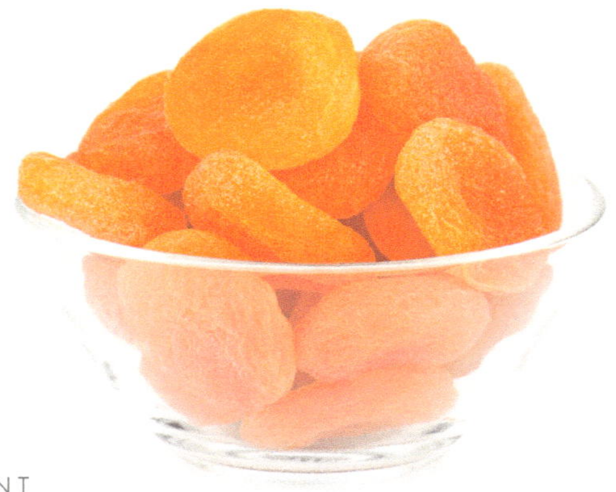

DINNER

BAKED SKINLESS CHICKEN BREAST AND RED CABBAGE WITH BAKED SWEET POTATO

- 6-ounce skinless chicken breast
- 1 cup raw red cabbage, shredded and sauteed in 2 teaspoons extra-virgin olive oil and ½ teaspoon of apple cider vinegar mixed with 1 garlic clove, minced
- ½ teaspoon black pepper (add to sauteed cabbage)
- 1 tablespoon lime juice (add to chicken or cabbage)
- 1 baked sweet potato

Season dinner meals with your choice and preference from the powdered condiments on the shopping list – salt-free garlic and onion powder are especially healthy options. Gradually eliminate seasoning food with salt as previously described in the Healthier Food Options section.

Meal Benefits

SKINLESS CHICKEN BREAST– contains lean protein and primarily unsaturated fats, which sustains healthy vascular function and helps reduce LDL (bad) cholesterol; provides vitamins B6 and B12, essential B-complex nutrients that reduce homocysteine levels (an amino acid that increases the risk of cardiovascular disease when elevated) and prevent anemia; also contributes potassium and magnesium, essential minerals which reduce blood pressure and therefore help prevent hypertension.

RED CABBAGE – contains vitamin C, a strong antioxidant that reduces oxygen free radicals, oxidative stress, and inflammation, which prevents vascular damage and injury; also provides soluble fiber that reduces LDL (bad) cholesterol, blood glucose, blood pressure, and body weight, and therefore helps prevent atherosclerosis, diabetes hypertension, and obesity.

GARLIC – contains allicin, a powerful antioxidant that reduces oxygen free radicals, oxidative stress, and inflammation, which prevents vascular damage and injury; also contains vitamin C and fiber, which reduces blood pressure, LDL (bad) cholesterol, blood

glucose, and body weight and therefore helps prevent hypertension, atherosclerosis, diabetes, and obesity.

LIME JUICE, FRESH – contains a high concentration of vitamin C, which is a powerful antioxidant that reduces oxygen free radicals, oxidative stress, and inflammation, which prevents vascular damage and injury; also provides potassium and magnesium, essential minerals that maintain proper water and electrolyte balance and therefore help reduce blood pressure and prevent hypertension.

BLACK PEPPER –contains the powerful antioxidant piperine that reduces oxygen free radicals, oxidative stress, and inflammation, which prevents vascular damage and injury; also contains potassium, calcium, and magnesium, essential minerals that lower blood pressure and LDL (bad) cholesterol levels and therefore help prevent hypertension and atherosclerosis.

SWEET POTATO – contains beta-carotene and vitamins B6 and C, antioxidants that reduce oxygen free radicals, oxidative stress, and inflammation, which prevents vascular damage and injury; provides calcium, potassium, and magnesium, essential minerals that sustain healthy vascular function and reduce blood pressure, which helps prevent hypertension; also contributes soluble fiber, which reduces LDL (bad) cholesterol, blood glucose, blood pressure, and body weight, and therefore also helps prevent atherosclerosis, diabetes, hypertension, and obesity.

OLIVE OIL – contains a high concentration of oleocanthal and vitamin E, powerful antioxidants that reduce oxygen free radicals, oxidative stress, and inflammation, which prevents vascular damage and injury; also provides a high concentration of monounsaturated fats, which lowers LDL (bad) cholesterol, increases HDL (good) cholesterol and therefore helps prevent atherosclerosis.

APPLE CIDER VINEGAR – contains polyphenols, powerful antioxidants that reduce oxygen free radicals, oxidative stress, and inflammation, which prevents vascular damage and injury; also contains acetic acid which lowers LDL (bad) cholesterol, blood pressure, blood glucose levels, and body weight and therefore helps prevent atherosclerosis, hypertension, diabetes, and obesity.

Dinner Calculations

Meal Total	Calories	Lean Protein	Complex Carbohydrates	Unsaturated Fat	Fiber
	385	41 gm	22 gm	14 gm	3 gm

HEART-HEALTHY SNACK

(eat at least several hours before going to sleep)

- ½ cup raspberries
- ½ apple

Snack Benefits

RASPBERRIES – contain anthocyanins, antioxidants that reduce oxygen free radicals, oxidative stress, and inflammation, which prevents vascular damage and injury; also provide a high concentration of soluble fiber, potassium, and manganese which reduces LDL (bad) cholesterol, blood glucose, body weight, and blood pressure and therefore helps prevent atherosclerosis, diabetes, obesity, and hypertension.

APPLE — contains a high concentration of vitamins C and B6, strong antioxidants that reduce oxygen free radicals, oxidative stress, and inflammation, which prevents vascular damage and injury; also contains magnesium and fiber, which reduces blood pressure, LDL (bad) cholesterol, blood glucose, and body weight and therefore helps prevent hypertension, atherosclerosis, diabetes, and obesity.

Snack Calculations

Snack Total	Calories	Lean Protein	Complex Carbohydrates	Unsaturated Fat	Fiber
	85	1 gm	22 gm	0 gm	6 gm

Daily Total Calculations

Daily Total	Calories	Lean Protein	Complex Carbohydrates	Unsaturated Fat	Fiber
	1822	78 gm	261 gm	60 gm	55 gm

BREAKFAST

NON-DAIRY YOGURT WITH GRANOLA AND FRESH FRUIT

- 12-ounce bowl of non-dairy yogurt (almond or oat-based)
- ½ cup classic whole grain rolled oats granola
- ½ orange
- ½ cup strawberries
- ½ apple

no added sugar or honey

Meal Benefits

NON-DIARY YOGURT – contains lean protein, which sustains healthy vascular function; contributes calcium and fiber, which reduces blood pressure, LDL (bad) cholesterol, blood glucose, and body weight and therefore helps prevent hypertension, atherosclerosis, diabetes, and obesity; provides healthy unsaturated fats, which lowers LDL (bad) cholesterol, increases HDL (good) cholesterol, and helps prevent atherosclerosis; also contains probiotics, which maintains healthy gut bacteria and intestinal health which reduces systemic inflammation that contributes to vascular damage and injury.

GRANOLA – contains a high concentration of soluble fiber, which reduces LDL (bad) cholesterol, blood glucose, blood pressure, and body weight and helps prevent atherosclerosis, diabetes, hypertension, and obesity; soluble fiber also promotes healthy gut bacteria and intestinal health which reduces systemic inflammation that contributes to vascular damage and injury; also contributes vitamin B1, manganese, and phytonutrients, potent antioxidants that reduce oxygen free radicals, oxidative stress, and inflammation, which prevents vascular damage and injury.

ORANGE – contains a high level of vitamin C, an antioxidant that reduces oxygen free radicals, oxidative stress, and inflammation, which prevents vascular damage and injury; also contains potassium and soluble fiber, which helps maintain proper water and electrolyte balance to reduce blood pressure, and lowers LDL (bad) cholesterol, blood glucose, and body weight, which helps prevent hypertension, atherosclerosis, diabetes, and obesity.

STRAWBERRIES – contain the antioxidants vitamin C, anthocyanins, and quercetin that reduce oxygen free radicals, oxidative stress, and inflammation, which prevents vascular damage and injury; also contribute soluble fiber, which reduces LDL (bad) cholesterol, blood glucose, blood pressure, and body weight and therefore helps prevent atherosclerosis, diabetes, hypertension, and obesity.

APPLE — contains a high concentration of vitamins C and B6, strong antioxidants that reduce oxygen free radicals, oxidative stress, and inflammation, which prevents vascular damage and injury; also contains magnesium and fiber, which reduces blood pressure, LDL (bad) cholesterol, blood glucose, and body weight and therefore helps prevent hypertension, atherosclerosis, diabetes, and obesity.

Breakfast Calculations

Meal Total	Calories	Lean Protein	Complex Carbohydrates	Unsaturated Fat	Fiber
	543	17 gm	58 gm	30 gm	21 gm

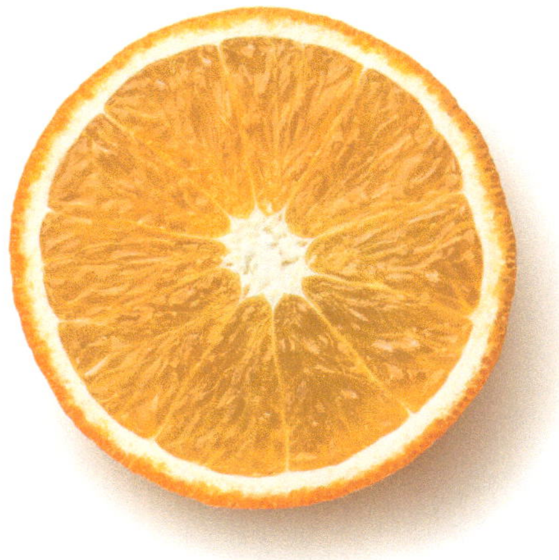

LUNCH

VEGETABLE SALAD WITH CHICKPEAS

- 2 cup baby spinach
- 1 cup chickpeas (*drain and rinse with cold water before eating*)
- ½ red bell pepper
- ½ red onion, sliced
- ½ avocado
- ½ cup of tomatoes

Olive oil vinaigrette – mix and add as salad dressing

- 2 tablespoons extra-virgin olive oil
- 1 tablespoon red wine vinegar
- 1 teaspoon paprika

Meal Benefits

SPINACH – contains phytonutrients and vitamin C, potent antioxidants that reduce oxygen free radicals, oxidative stress, and inflammation, which prevents vascular damage and injury; also contributes vitamin D, calcium, and fiber, which reduces blood pressure, LDL (bad) cholesterol, blood glucose, and body weight and therefore helps prevent hypertension, atherosclerosis, diabetes, and obesity.

CHICKPEAS — contain lean protein, iron, and soluble fiber, which sustains healthy vascular function, prevents anemia, reduces blood pressure, LDL (bad) cholesterol, blood glucose, and body weight, and therefore helps prevent atherosclerosis, hypertension, diabetes, and obesity.

RED BELL PEPPER – contains high levels of the antioxidants vitamins C and B6 that reduce oxygen free radicals, oxidative stress, and inflammation, which prevents vascular damage and injury; also contributes potassium and soluble fiber, which reduces blood pressure, LDL (bad) cholesterol, blood

glucose, and body weight and therefore helps prevent hypertension, atherosclerosis, diabetes, and obesity.

RED ONIONS – contain the powerful antioxidants quercetin and vitamin C that reduce oxygen free radicals, oxidative stress, and inflammation, which prevents vascular damage and injury; also contribute calcium and fiber, which reduces blood pressure, LDL (bad) cholesterol, blood glucose, and body weight and therefore helps prevent hypertension, atherosclerosis, diabetes, and obesity.

AVOCADO – contains healthy monounsaturated fats, which lowers LDL (bad) cholesterol, increases HDL (good) cholesterol, and therefore helps prevent atherosclerosis; contributes the antioxidants vitamins C and E, and copper that reduce oxygen free radicals, oxidative stress, and inflammation, which prevents vascular damage and injury; also provides manganese which reduces blood pressure and therefore helps prevent hypertension.

TOMATOES – contain lycopene and vitamins B, C, and E, powerful antioxidants that reduce oxygen free radicals, oxidative stress, and inflammation, which prevents vascular damage and injury; also contain a high concentration of potassium, which lowers blood pressure to prevent hypertension.

OLIVE OIL – contains a high concentration of oleocanthal and vitamin E, powerful antioxidants that reduce oxygen free radicals, oxidative stress, and inflammation, which prevents vascular damage and injury; also provides a high concentration of monounsaturated fats, which lowers LDL (bad) cholesterol, increases HDL (good) cholesterol and therefore helps prevent atherosclerosis.

RED WINE VINEGAR – contains polyphenols, powerful antioxidants that reduce oxygen free radicals, oxidative stress, and inflammation, which prevents vascular damage and injury; also contains acetic acid which lowers LDL (bad) cholesterol, blood pressure, blood glucose levels, and body weight and therefore helps prevent atherosclerosis, hypertension, diabetes, and obesity.

PAPRIKA –contains carotenoids and vitamins A, B6, C, and E, all powerful antioxidants that reduce oxygen free radicals, oxidative stress, and inflammation, which prevents vascular damage and injury; also provides potassium, which lowers blood pressure and therefore helps prevent hypertension.

Lunch Calculations

Meal Total	Calories	Lean Protein	Complex Carbohydrates	Unsaturated Fat	Fiber
	641	17 gm	60 gm	41 gm	22 gm

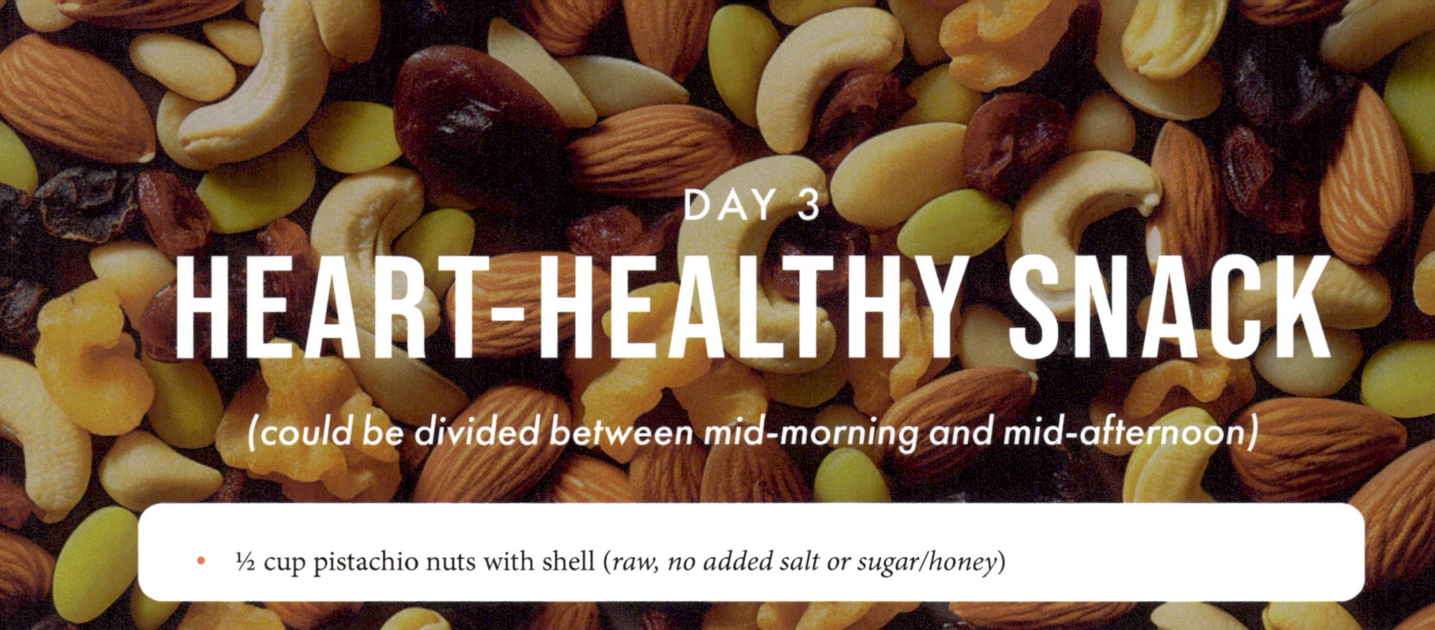

HEART-HEALTHY SNACK

(could be divided between mid-morning and mid-afternoon)

- ½ cup pistachio nuts with shell (*raw, no added salt or sugar/honey*)

Snack Benefits

PISTACHIOS – lower-calorie nuts that provide an excellent source of phosphorous and vitamins B1 and B6, which have significant antioxidant and anti-inflammatory properties that reduce oxygen free radicals, oxidative stress, and inflammation, helping to prevent vascular damage and injury; also contain high levels of lean protein, unsaturated fats, and fiber, which sustains healthy vascular function and reduces LDL (bad) cholesterol, blood pressure, blood glucose, and body weight.

Snack Calculations

Snack Total	Calories	Lean Protein	Complex Carbohydrates	Unsaturated Fat	Fiber
	160	6 gm	8 gm	13 gm	3 gm

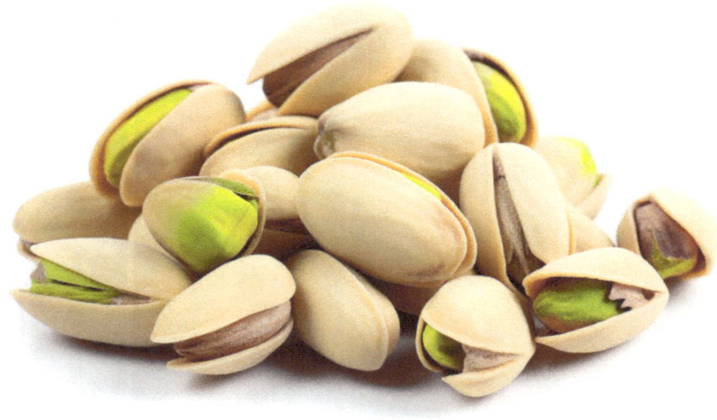

DINNER

SAUTEED COD LOIN FILET AND SAUTEED TOMATOES, ONIONS, AND PEPPERS WITH BROWN RICE

- 6-ounce cod loin filet
- 1 tablespoon extra-virgin olive oil (use to sauté cod loin filet and vegetables)
- 1 cup tomatoes
- ½ sliced red onion
- ½ green bell pepper
- 1 garlic clove, minced
- 1 teaspoon oregano
- ½ teaspoon black pepper
- ½ cup of brown rice

Season dinner meals with your choice and preference from the powdered condiments on the shopping list – salt-free garlic and onion powder are especially healthy options. Gradually eliminate seasoning food with salt as previously described in the Healthier Food Options section.

Meal Benefits

COD – contains lean protein and high concentrations of vitamins B6 and B12, which helps maintain healthy vascular function, prevents anemia, and therefore reduces the risk of vascular damage and injury; provides a high concentration of polyunsaturated fats called omega-3 fatty acids, which lowers LDL (bad) cholesterol, increases HDL (good) cholesterol and therefore helps prevent atherosclerosis; also contributes phosphorus, an antioxidant that reduces oxygen free radicals, oxidative stress, and inflammation, which prevents vascular damage and injury.

TOMATOES – contain lycopene and vitamins B, C, and E, powerful antioxidants that reduce oxygen free radicals, oxidative stress, and inflammation, which prevents vascular damage and injury; also contain a high concentration of potassium, which lowers blood pressure to prevent hypertension.

RED ONIONS – contain the powerful antioxidants quercetin and vitamin C that reduce oxygen free radicals, oxidative stress, and inflammation, which prevents vascular damage and injury; also contribute calcium and fiber, which reduces blood pressure, LDL (bad) cholesterol, blood glucose, and body weight and therefore helps prevent hypertension, atherosclerosis, diabetes, and obesity.

GREEN BELL PEPPER – contains high levels of the antioxidants vitamins C and B6 that reduce oxygen free radicals, oxidative stress, and inflammation, which prevents vascular damage and injury; also contributes potassium and soluble fiber, which reduces blood pressure, LDL (bad) cholesterol, blood glucose, and body weight and therefore helps prevent hypertension, atherosclerosis, diabetes, and obesity.

GARLIC – contains allicin, a powerful antioxidant that reduces oxygen free radicals, oxidative stress, and inflammation, which prevents vascular damage and injury; also contains vitamin C and fiber, which reduces blood pressure, LDL (bad) cholesterol, blood glucose, and body weight and therefore helps prevent hypertension, atherosclerosis, diabetes, and obesity.

OLIVE OIL – contains a high concentration of oleocanthal and vitamin E, powerful antioxidants that reduce oxygen free radicals, oxidative stress, and inflammation, which prevents vascular damage and injury; also provides a high concentration of monounsaturated fats, which lowers LDL (bad) cholesterol, increases HDL (good) cholesterol and therefore helps prevent atherosclerosis.

BROWN RICE (WHOLE GRAIN, MOST OF THE VITAMINS AND MINERALS ARE IN THE TWO OUTER LAYERS OF RICE) – a complex carbohydrate low on the glycemic index (an index that measures how much a food increases your blood sugar levels) and rich in lean protein, calcium, iron, magnesium, and soluble fiber, which sustains healthy vascular function and reduces LDL (bad) cholesterol, blood glucose, and body weight, and therefore helps prevent hypertension, atherosclerosis, diabetes, and obesity; also contains flavonoid antioxidants that reduce oxygen free radicals, oxidative stress, and inflammation, which prevents vascular damage and injury.

OREGANO – contains a high concentration of polyphenol antioxidants, including carvacrol, that reduce oxygen free radicals, oxidative stress, and inflammation, which prevents vascular damage and injury; also provides high levels of calcium, which is essential to normal cardiac and vascular function and helps reduce blood pressure and therefore prevent hypertension.

BLACK PEPPER –contains the powerful antioxidant piperine that reduces oxygen free radicals, oxidative stress, and inflammation, which prevents vascular damage and injury; also contains potassium, calcium, and magnesium, essential minerals that lower blood pressure and LDL (bad) cholesterol levels and therefore help prevent hypertension and atherosclerosis.

Dinner Calculations

Meal Total	Calories	Lean Protein	Complex Carbohydrates	Unsaturated Fat	Fiber
	436	46 gm	29 gm	16 gm	4 gm

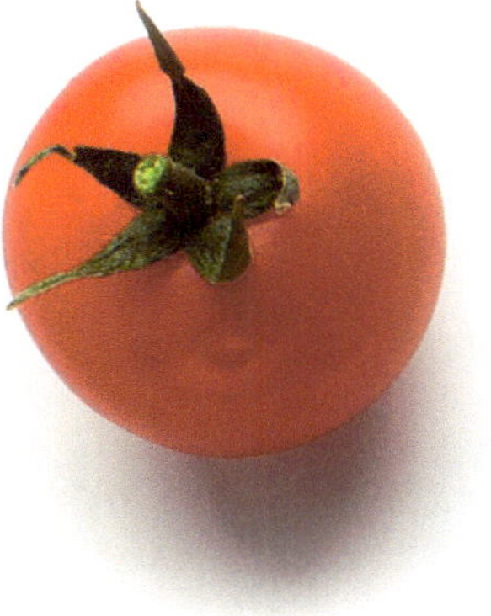

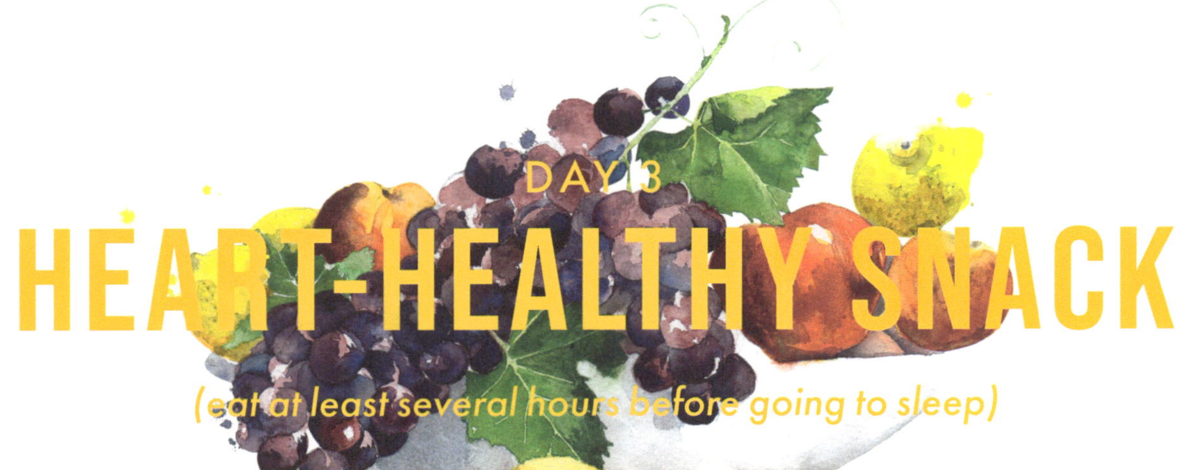

- ½ cup red grapes
- ½ banana

Snack Benefits

RED GRAPES – contain a high concentration of potassium, which helps maintain proper water and electrolyte balance to sustain normal blood pressure and prevent hypertension; also contain resveratrol and vitamin C, strong antioxidants that reduce oxygen free radicals, oxidative stress, and inflammation, which prevents vascular damage and injury.

BANANA – contains vitamin C, an antioxidant that reduces oxygen free radicals, oxidative stress, and inflammation, which prevents vascular damage and injury; also contains a high concentration of potassium and fiber, which helps prevent hypertension, atherosclerosis, diabetes, and obesity by reducing blood pressure, LDL (bad) cholesterol, blood glucose, and body weight.

Snack Calculations

Snack Total	Calories	Lean Protein	Complex Carbohydrates	Unsaturated Fat	Fiber
	113	2 gm	28 gm	0 gm	3 gm

Daily Total Calculations

Daily Total	Calories	Lean Protein	Complex Carbohydrates	Unsaturated Fat	Fiber
	1893	88 gm	183 gm	100 gm	53 gm

BREAKFAST

OATMEAL WITH FRESH FRUIT

- 12-ounce bowl of traditional old-fashioned oatmeal cooked with 1½ cups unsweetened, unflavored non-dairy milk (almond or oat-based)
- ½ cup raspberries
- ½ banana
- ½ apple

no added sugar or honey

Meal Benefits

OATMEAL – contains a high concentration of the soluble fiber beta-glucan, which reduces LDL (bad) cholesterol, blood glucose, blood pressure, and body weight and therefore helps prevent atherosclerosis, diabetes, hypertension, and obesity; beta-glucan also promotes healthy gut bacteria and intestinal health which reduces systemic inflammation that contributes to vascular damage and injury; also contributes vitamin B1, manganese, and phytonutrients, potent antioxidants that reduce oxygen free radicals, oxidative stress, and inflammation, which prevents vascular damage and injury.

NON-DAIRY MILK (ALMOND OR OAT-BASED) – contains no cholesterol, and lower total calories and sugar than dairy milk, reducing the risk of atherosclerosis and diabetes; also contributes lean protein and calcium, two nutrients that help sustain healthy vascular function, regulate normal blood pressure, and prevent hypertension.

RASPBERRIES – contain anthocyanins, antioxidants that reduce oxygen free radicals, oxidative stress, and inflammation, which prevents vascular damage and injury; also provide a high concentration of soluble fiber, potassium, and manganese which reduces LDL (bad) cholesterol, blood glucose, body weight, and blood pressure and therefore helps prevent atherosclerosis, diabetes, obesity, and hypertension.

BANANA – contains vitamin C, an antioxidant that reduces oxygen free radicals, oxidative stress, and inflammation, which prevents vascular damage and injury; also contains a high concentration of potassium and fiber, which helps prevent hypertension, atherosclerosis, diabetes, and obesity by reducing blood pressure, LDL (bad) cholesterol, blood glucose, and body weight.

APPLE — contains a high concentration of vitamins C and B6, strong antioxidants that reduce oxygen free radicals, oxidative stress, and inflammation, which prevents vascular damage and injury; also contains magnesium and fiber, which reduces blood pressure, LDL (bad) cholesterol, blood glucose, and body weight and therefore helps prevent hypertension, atherosclerosis, diabetes, and obesity.

Breakfast Calculations

Meal Total	Calories	Lean Protein	Complex Carbohydrates	Unsaturated Fat	Fiber
	560	16 gm	112 gm	9 gm	18 gm

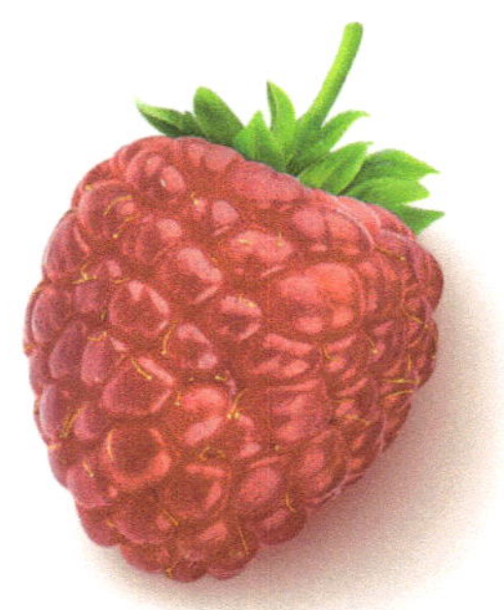

LUNCH

VEGETABLE SALAD WITH KIDNEY BEANS

- 2 cups kale
- 1 cup kidney beans (*drain and rinse with cold water before eating*)
- 1 garlic clove, chopped
- ½ cup uncooked broccoli
- ½ cup carrots
- ½ cucumber

Olive oil vinaigrette – mix and add as salad dressing

- 2 tablespoons extra-virgin olive oil
- 1 tablespoon apple wine vinegar
- 1 teaspoon cumin

Meal Benefits

KALE – contains vitamin C and phytonutrients, antioxidants that reduce oxygen free radicals, oxidative stress, and inflammation, which prevents vascular damage and injury; also contains vitamin D, calcium, and fiber, which reduces blood pressure, LDL (bad) cholesterol, blood glucose, and body weight and therefore helps prevent hypertension, atherosclerosis, diabetes, and obesity.

KIDNEY BEANS — contain lean protein, iron, and soluble fiber, which sustains healthy vascular function, prevents anemia, reduces blood pressure, LDL (bad) cholesterol, blood glucose, and body weight, and therefore helps prevent hypertension, atherosclerosis, diabetes, and obesity.

GARLIC – contains allicin, a powerful antioxidant that reduces oxygen free radicals, oxidative stress, and inflammation, which prevents vascular damage and injury; also contains vitamin C and fiber, which reduces blood pressure, LDL (bad) cholesterol, blood glucose, and body weight and therefore helps prevent hypertension, atherosclerosis, diabetes, and obesity.

BROCCOLI – contains flavonoids, carotenoids including lutein and beta-carotene, and vitamin C, which are powerful antioxidants that reduce oxygen free radicals, oxidative stress, and inflammation, which prevents vascular damage and injury; also contains a high concentration of soluble fiber, which reduces LDL (bad) cholesterol, blood glucose, blood pressure, and body weight, and therefore helps prevent atherosclerosis, diabetes, hypertension, and obesity.

CARROTS – contain vitamins A and C, and beta-carotene, strong antioxidants that reduce oxygen free radicals, oxidative stress, and inflammation, which prevents vascular damage and injury; also contribute fiber, which reduces LDL (bad) cholesterol, blood glucose, blood pressure, and body weight and therefore helps prevent atherosclerosis, diabetes, hypertension, and obesity.

CUCUMBER UNPEELED (PEELING REDUCES THE AMOUNT OF FIBER, VITAMINS, AND MINERALS) – contains vitamin C, a strong antioxidant that reduces oxygen free radicals, oxidative stress, and inflammation, which prevents vascular damage and injury; provides magnesium and potassium, essential minerals that help maintain proper water and electrolyte balance to sustain normal blood pressure and prevent hypertension; also

provides fiber, which reduces LDL (bad) cholesterol, blood glucose, and body weight, and therefore helps prevent atherosclerosis, diabetes, and obesity.

OLIVE OIL – contains a high concentration of oleocanthal and vitamin E, powerful antioxidants that reduce oxygen free radicals, oxidative stress, and inflammation, which prevents vascular damage and injury; also provides a high concentration of monounsaturated fats, which lowers LDL (bad) cholesterol, increases HDL (good) cholesterol and therefore helps prevent atherosclerosis.

APPLE WINE VINEGAR – contains polyphenols, powerful antioxidants that reduce oxygen free radicals, oxidative stress, and inflammation, which prevents vascular damage and injury; also contains acetic acid which lowers LDL (bad) cholesterol, blood pressure, blood glucose levels, and body weight and therefore helps prevent atherosclerosis, hypertension, diabetes, and obesity.

CUMIN – contains polyphenols and flavonoids, antioxidants that reduce oxygen free radicals, oxidative stress, and inflammation, which prevents vascular damage and injury; also contributes high levels of iron, which prevents anemia and sustains healthy vascular function, and therefore helps prevent atherosclerosis and hypertension.

Lunch Calculations

Meal Total	Calories	Lean Protein	Complex Carbohydrates	Unsaturated Fat	Fiber
	428	11 gm	36 gm	29 gm	13 gm

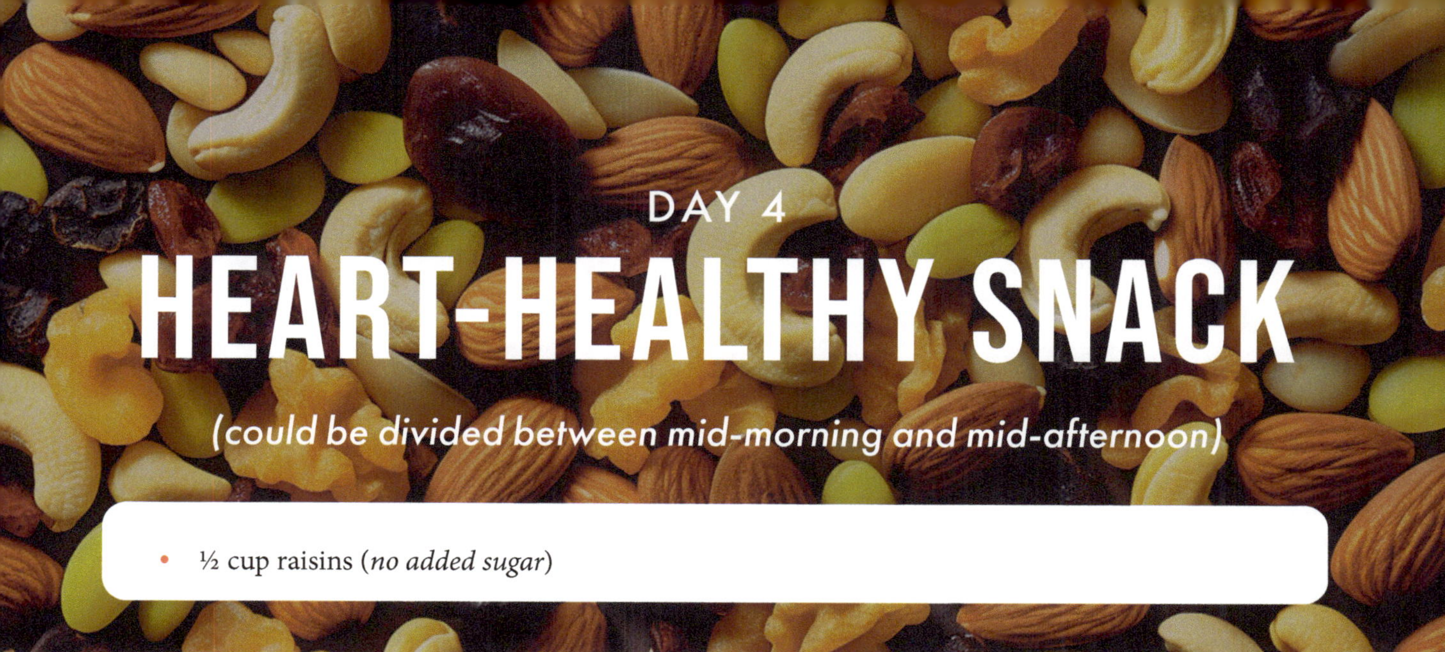

- ½ cup raisins (*no added sugar*)

Snack Benefits

RAISINS – contain a high concentration of phytonutrients, strong antioxidants that reduce oxygen free radicals, oxidative stress, and inflammation, which prevents vascular damage and injury; contain a high concentration of potassium, which lowers blood pressure to prevent hypertension; also provide a good source of fiber, which reduces LDL (bad) cholesterol, blood glucose, and body weight.

Snack Calculations

Snack Total	Calories	Lean Protein	Complex Carbohydrates	Unsaturated Fat	Fiber
	240	2 gm	62 gm	0 gm	4 gm

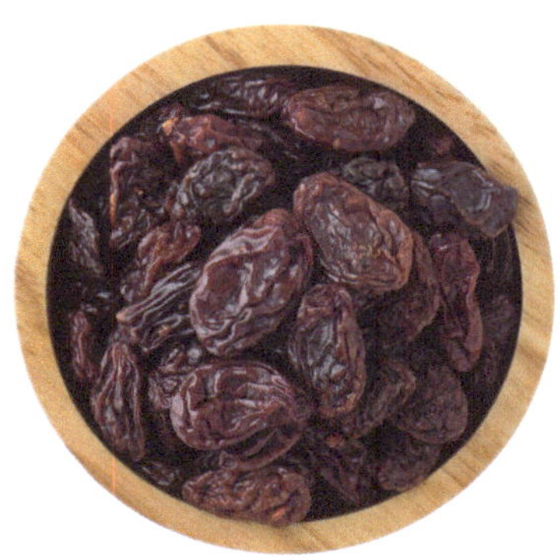

DINNER

SAUTEED TILAPIA AND AVOCADO, TOMATO, AND RED ONION SALAD WITH SWEET POTATO

- 8-ounce sauteed tilapia filet
- 1 tablespoon of extra-virgin olive oil (use to sauté tilapia)
- ½ avocado
- ½ cup tomatoes
- ½ red onion, sliced
- 1 tablespoon fresh lime juice (add to vegetable salad)
- 1 mashed sweet potato

Season dinner meals with your choice and preference from the powdered condiments on the shopping list – salt-free garlic and onion powder are especially healthy options. Gradually eliminate seasoning food with salt as previously described in the Healthier Food Options section.

Meal Benefits

TILAPIA – contains high concentrations of vitamin B6, a powerful antioxidant that reduces oxygen free radicals, oxidative stress, and inflammation, which prevents vascular damage and injury; provides a high concentration of polyunsaturated fats called omega-3 fatty acids, which lowers LDL (bad) cholesterol, increases HDL (good) cholesterol and therefore helps prevent atherosclerosis; also contributes vitamin D, potassium, and magnesium, which lowers blood pressure and LDL (bad) cholesterol levels and therefore helps prevent hypertension and atherosclerosis.

AVOCADO – contains healthy monounsaturated fats, which lowers LDL (bad) cholesterol, increases HDL (good) cholesterol, and therefore helps prevent atherosclerosis; contributes the antioxidants vitamins C and E, and copper that reduce oxygen free radicals, oxidative stress, and inflammation, which prevents vascular damage and injury; also provides manganese which reduces blood pressure and therefore helps prevent hypertension.

TOMATOES – contain lycopene and vitamins B, C, and E, powerful antioxidants that reduce oxygen free radicals, oxidative stress, and inflammation, which prevents vascular damage and injury; also contain a high concentration of potassium, which lowers blood pressure to prevent hypertension.

RED ONIONS – contain the powerful antioxidants quercetin and vitamin C that reduce oxygen free radicals, oxidative stress, and inflammation, which prevents vascular damage and injury; also contribute calcium and fiber, which reduces blood pressure, LDL (bad) cholesterol, blood glucose, and body weight and therefore helps prevent hypertension, atherosclerosis, diabetes, and obesity.

LIME JUICE, FRESH – contains a high concentration of vitamin C, which is a powerful antioxidant that reduces oxygen free radicals, oxidative stress, and inflammation, which prevents vascular damage and injury; also provides potassium and magnesium, essential minerals that maintain proper water and electrolyte balance and therefore help reduce blood pressure and prevent hypertension.

OLIVE OIL – contains a high concentration of oleocanthal and vitamin E, powerful antioxidants that reduce oxygen free radicals, oxidative stress, and inflammation, which prevents vascular damage and injury; also provides a high concentration of monounsaturated fats, which lowers LDL (bad) cholesterol, increases HDL (good) cholesterol and therefore helps prevent atherosclerosis.

SWEET POTATO – contains beta-carotene and vitamins B6 and C, antioxidants that reduce oxygen free radicals, oxidative stress, and inflammation, which prevents vascular damage and injury; provides calcium, potassium, and magnesium, essential minerals that sustain healthy vascular function and reduce blood pressure, which helps prevent hypertension; also contributes soluble fiber, which reduces LDL (bad) cholesterol, blood glucose, blood pressure, and body weight, and therefore helps prevent atherosclerosis, diabetes, hypertension, and obesity.

Dinner Calculations

Meal Total	Calories	Lean Protein	Complex Carbohydrates	Unsaturated Fat	Fiber
	595	51 gm	38 gm	29 gm	10 gm

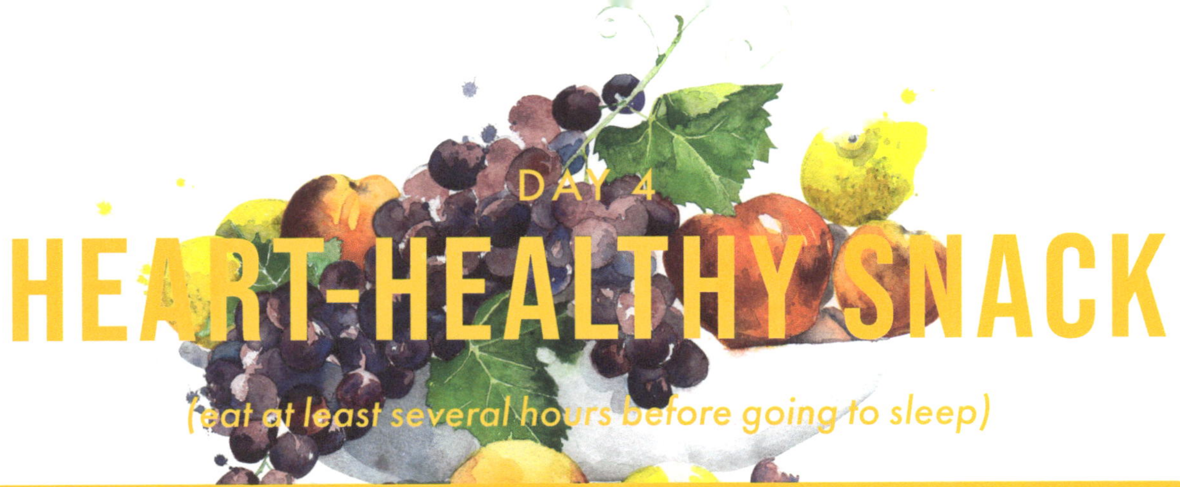

HEART-HEALTHY SNACK

(eat at least several hours before going to sleep)

- ½ cup blueberries
- ½ orange

Snack Benefits

BLUEBERRIES – contain the highest concentration of the antioxidants anthocyanins among all fresh fruits, reducing oxygen free radicals, oxidative stress, and inflammation, which prevents vascular damage and injury; also contain a high concentration of vitamin C and soluble fiber, which reduces blood pressure, LDL (bad) cholesterol, blood glucose, and body weight and therefore helps prevent hypertension, atherosclerosis, diabetes, and obesity.

ORANGE – contains a high level of vitamin C, an antioxidant that reduces oxygen free radicals, oxidative stress, and inflammation, which prevents vascular damage and injury; also contains potassium and soluble fiber, which helps maintain proper water and electrolyte balance to reduce blood pressure, and lowers LDL (bad) cholesterol, blood glucose, and body weight, which helps prevent hypertension, atherosclerosis, diabetes, and obesity.

Snack Calculations

Snack Total	Calories	Lean Protein	Complex Carbohydrates	Unsaturated Fat	Fiber
	71	2 gm	18 gm	0 gm	4 gm

Daily Total Calculations

Daily Total	Calories	Lean Protein	Complex Carbohydrates	Unsaturated Fat	Fiber
	1893	83 gm	267 gm	67 gm	49 gm

BREAKFAST

WHOLE GRAIN SHREDDED WHEAT OR BRAN HIGH-FIBER CEREAL WITH FRESH FRUIT

- 12-ounce bowl of whole grain shredded wheat or bran high-fiber cereal
- 1½ cups unsweetened, unflavored non-dairy milk (almond or oat-based)
- ½ cup raspberries
- ½ orange
- ½ cup of blueberries

no added sugar or honey

Meal Benefits

WHOLE GRAIN SHREDDED WHEAT OR BRAN HIGH-FIBER CEREAL – contains a high concentration of fiber, which reduces LDL (bad) cholesterol, blood glucose, blood pressure, and body weight and therefore helps prevent atherosclerosis, diabetes, hypertension, and obesity; fiber also promotes healthy gut bacteria and intestinal health which reduces systemic inflammation that contributes to vascular damage and injury; also an excellent source of phosphorous which has significant antioxidant properties that reduce oxygen free radicals, oxidative stress, and inflammation, helping to prevent atherosclerosis.

NON-DAIRY MILK (ALMOND OR OAT-BASED) – contains no cholesterol, and lower total calories and sugar than dairy milk, reducing the risk of atherosclerosis and diabetes; also contributes lean protein and calcium, two nutrients that help sustain healthy vascular function, regulate normal blood pressure, and prevent hypertension.

RASPBERRIES – contain anthocyanins, antioxidants that reduce oxygen free radicals, oxidative stress, and inflammation, which prevents vascular damage and injury; also provide a high concentration of soluble fiber, potassium, and manganese which reduce LDL (bad) cholesterol, blood glucose, body weight, and blood pressure and therefore help prevent atherosclerosis, diabetes, obesity, and hypertension.

ORANGE – contains a high level of vitamin C, an antioxidant that reduces oxygen free radicals, oxidative stress, and inflammation, which prevents vascular damage and injury; also contains potassium and soluble fiber, which helps maintain proper water and electrolyte balance to reduce blood pressure, and lowers LDL (bad) cholesterol, blood glucose, and body weight, which helps prevent hypertension, atherosclerosis, diabetes, and obesity.

BLUEBERRIES – contain the highest concentration of the antioxidants anthocyanins among all fresh fruits, reducing oxygen free radicals, oxidative stress, and inflammation, which prevents vascular damage and injury; also contain a high concentration of vitamin C and soluble fiber, which reduces blood pressure, LDL (bad) cholesterol, blood glucose, and body weight and therefore helps prevent hypertension, atherosclerosis, diabetes, and obesity.

Breakfast Calculations

Meal Total	Calories	Lean Protein	Complex Carbohydrates	Unsaturated Fat	Fiber
	455	15 gm	97 gm	5 gm	20 gm

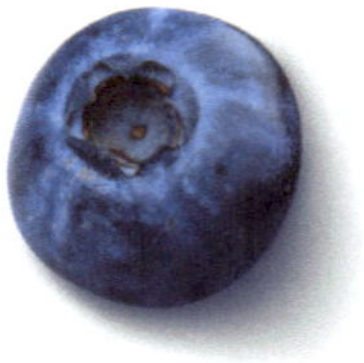

LUNCH

VEGETABLE SALAD WITH BLACK BEANS

- 2 cups spinach
- 1 cup black beans (*drain and rinse with cold water before eating*)
- ½ yellow bell pepper
- ½ cup tomatoes
- ½ red onion, sliced
- ½ avocado

Olive oil vinaigrette – mix and add as salad dressing

- 2 tablespoons extra-virgin olive oil
- 1 tablespoon red wine vinegar
- 1 teaspoon cayenne pepper

Meal Benefits

SPINACH – contains phytonutrients and vitamin C, potent antioxidants that reduce oxygen free radicals, oxidative stress, and inflammation, which prevents vascular damage and injury; also contributes vitamin D, calcium, and fiber, which reduces blood pressure, LDL (bad) cholesterol, blood glucose, and body weight and therefore helps prevent hypertension, atherosclerosis, diabetes, and obesity.

BLACK BEANS — contain lean protein, iron, and soluble fiber, which sustains healthy vascular function, prevents anemia, reduces blood pressure, LDL (bad) cholesterol, blood glucose, and body weight, and therefore helps prevent atherosclerosis, hypertension, diabetes, and obesity.

YELLOW BELL PEPPER – contains high levels of the antioxidants vitamins C and B6 that reduce oxygen free radicals, oxidative stress, and inflammation, which prevents vascular damage and injury; also contributes potassium and soluble fiber, which reduces blood pressure, LDL (bad) cholesterol, blood

glucose, and body weight and therefore helps prevent hypertension, atherosclerosis, diabetes, and obesity.

TOMATOES – contain lycopene and vitamins B, C, and E, powerful antioxidants that reduce oxygen free radicals, oxidative stress, and inflammation, which prevents vascular damage and injury; also contain a high concentration of potassium, which lowers blood pressure to prevent hypertension.

RED ONIONS – contain the powerful antioxidants quercetin and vitamin C that reduce oxygen free radicals, oxidative stress, and inflammation, which prevents vascular damage and injury; also contribute calcium and fiber, which reduces blood pressure, LDL (bad) cholesterol, blood glucose, and body weight and therefore helps prevent hypertension, atherosclerosis, diabetes, and obesity.

AVOCADO – contains healthy monounsaturated fats, which lowers LDL (bad) cholesterol, increases HDL (good) cholesterol, and therefore helps prevent atherosclerosis; contributes the antioxidants vitamins C and E, and copper that reduce oxygen free radicals, oxidative stress, and inflammation, which prevents vascular damage and injury; also provides manganese which reduces blood pressure and therefore helps prevent hypertension.

OLIVE OIL – contains a high concentration of oleocanthal and vitamin E, powerful antioxidants that reduce oxygen free radicals, oxidative stress, and inflammation, which prevents vascular damage and injury; also provides a high concentration of monounsaturated fats, which lowers LDL (bad) cholesterol, increases HDL (good) cholesterol and therefore helps prevent atherosclerosis.

RED WINE VINEGAR – contains polyphenols, powerful antioxidants that reduce oxygen free radicals, oxidative stress, and inflammation, which prevents vascular damage and injury; also contains acetic acid which lowers LDL (bad) cholesterol, blood pressure, blood glucose levels, and body weight and therefore helps prevent atherosclerosis, hypertension, diabetes, and obesity.

CAYENNE PEPPER– contains capsaicin, a powerful antioxidant that reduces oxygen free radicals, oxidative stress, and inflammation, which prevents vascular damage and injury; also provides potassium and manganese, essential minerals which lower blood pressure and LDL (bad) cholesterol and therefore help prevent hypertension and atherosclerosis.

Lunch Calculations

Meal Total	Calories	Lean Protein	Complex Carbohydrates	Unsaturated Fat	Fiber
	643	19 gm	60 gm	39 gm	27 gm

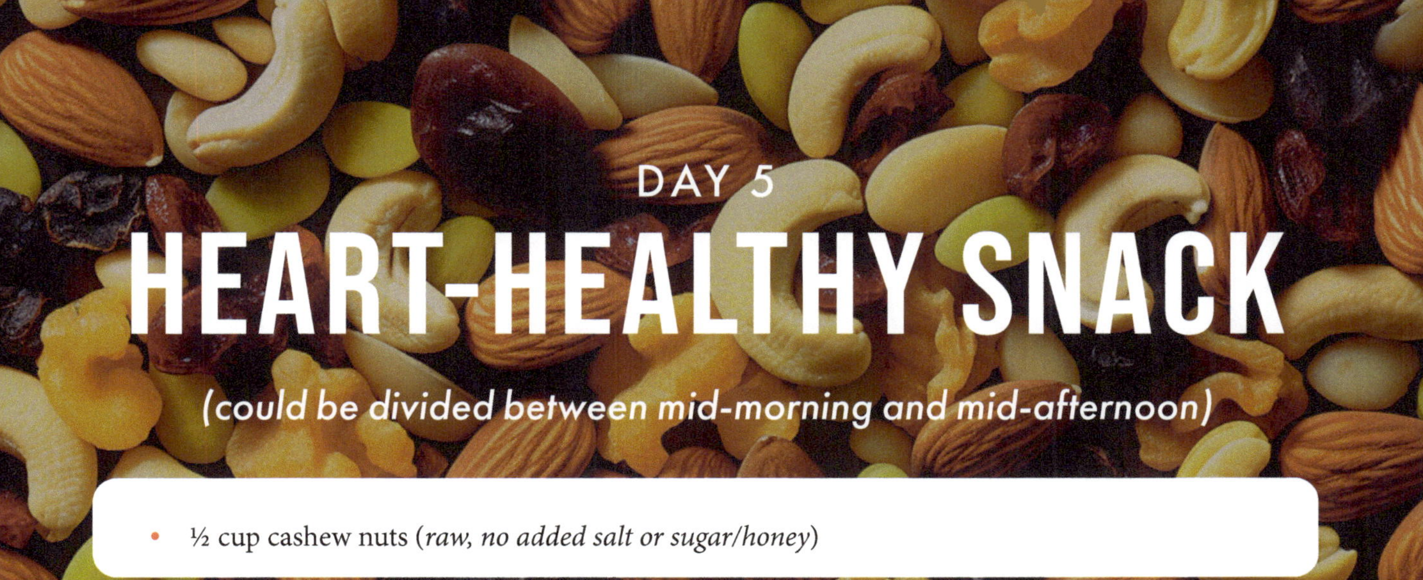

Snack Benefits

CASHEWS: an excellent source of potassium, magnesium, and iron, essential minerals that reduce blood pressure, LDL (bad) cholesterol, and prevent anemia, which helps prevent hypertension and atherosclerosis; contain high levels of lean protein, unsaturated fats, and fiber, which sustains healthy vascular function, reduces LDL (bad) cholesterol, blood glucose, and body weight; also rich in carotenoids and polyphenols, antioxidants that reduce oxygen free radicals, oxidative stress, and inflammation, which prevents vascular damage and injury.

Snack Calculations

Snack Total	Calories	Lean Protein	Complex Carbohydrates	Unsaturated Fat	Fiber
	320	10 gm	16 gm	24 gm	2 gm

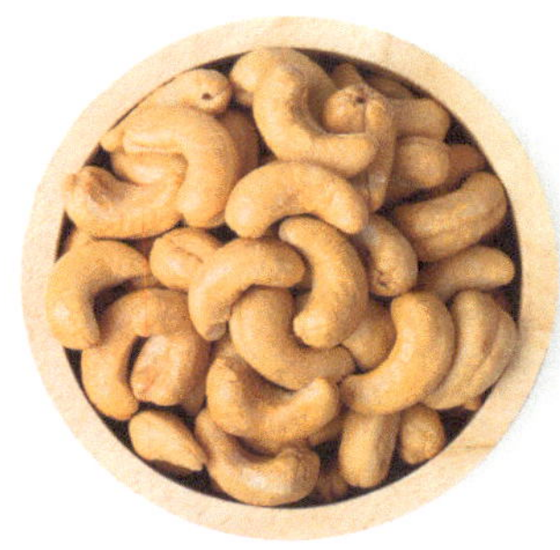

DINNER

BAKED SKINLESS CHICKEN BREAST AND VEGETABLE MIX WITH BROWN RICE

- 6 ounces of skinless chicken breast
- ½ cup chopped red onion
- 1 garlic clove, chopped
- ½ cup diced carrots
- ½ yellow bell pepper
- ½ cup brown rice

Season dinner meals with your choice and preference from the powdered condiments on the shopping list – salt-free garlic and onion powder are especially healthy options. Gradually eliminate seasoning food with salt as previously described in the Healthier Food Options section.

Meal Benefits

SKINLESS CHICKEN BREAST– contains lean protein and primarily unsaturated fats, which sustains healthy vascular function and helps reduce LDL (bad) cholesterol; provides vitamins B6 and B12, essential B-complex nutrients that reduce homocysteine levels (an amino acid that increases the risk of cardiovascular diseases when elevated) and prevent anemia; also contributes potassium and magnesium, essential minerals which reduce blood pressure and therefore help prevent hypertension.

CARROTS – contain vitamins A and C, and beta-carotene, strong antioxidants that reduce oxygen free radicals, oxidative stress, and inflammation, which prevents vascular damage and injury; also contribute fiber, which reduces LDL (bad) cholesterol, blood glucose, blood pressure, and body weight and therefore helps prevent atherosclerosis, diabetes, hypertension, and obesity.

RED ONIONS – contain the powerful antioxidants quercetin and vitamin C that reduce oxygen free radicals, oxidative stress, and inflammation, which prevents vascular damage and injury; also contribute calcium and fiber, which reduces blood pressure, LDL (bad) cholesterol, blood glucose, and body weight and therefore helps prevent hypertension, atherosclerosis, diabetes, and obesity.

YELLOW BELL PEPPER – contains high levels of the antioxidants vitamins C and B6 that reduce oxygen free radicals, oxidative stress, and inflammation, which prevents vascular damage and injury; also contributes potassium and soluble fiber, which reduces blood pressure, LDL (bad) cholesterol, blood glucose, and body weight and therefore helps prevent hypertension, atherosclerosis, diabetes, and obesity.

GARLIC – contains allicin, a powerful antioxidant that reduces oxygen free radicals, oxidative stress, and inflammation, which prevents vascular damage

and injury; also contains vitamin C and fiber, which reduces blood pressure, LDL (bad) cholesterol, blood glucose, and body weight and therefore helps prevent hypertension, atherosclerosis, diabetes, and obesity.

BROWN RICE (WHOLE GRAIN, MOST OF THE VITAMINS AND MINERALS ARE IN THE TWO OUTER LAYERS OF RICE) – a complex carbohydrate low on the glycemic index (an index that measures how much a food increases your blood sugar levels) and rich in lean protein, calcium, iron, magnesium, and soluble fiber, which sustains healthy vascular function and reduces LDL (bad) cholesterol, blood glucose, and body weight, and therefore helps prevent hypertension, atherosclerosis, diabetes, and obesity; also contains flavonoid antioxidants that reduce oxygen free radicals, oxidative stress, and inflammation, which prevents vascular damage and injury.

Dinner Calculations

Meal Total	Calories	Lean Protein	Complex Carbohydrates	Unsaturated Fat	Fiber
	384	43 gm	42 gm	4 gm	8 gm

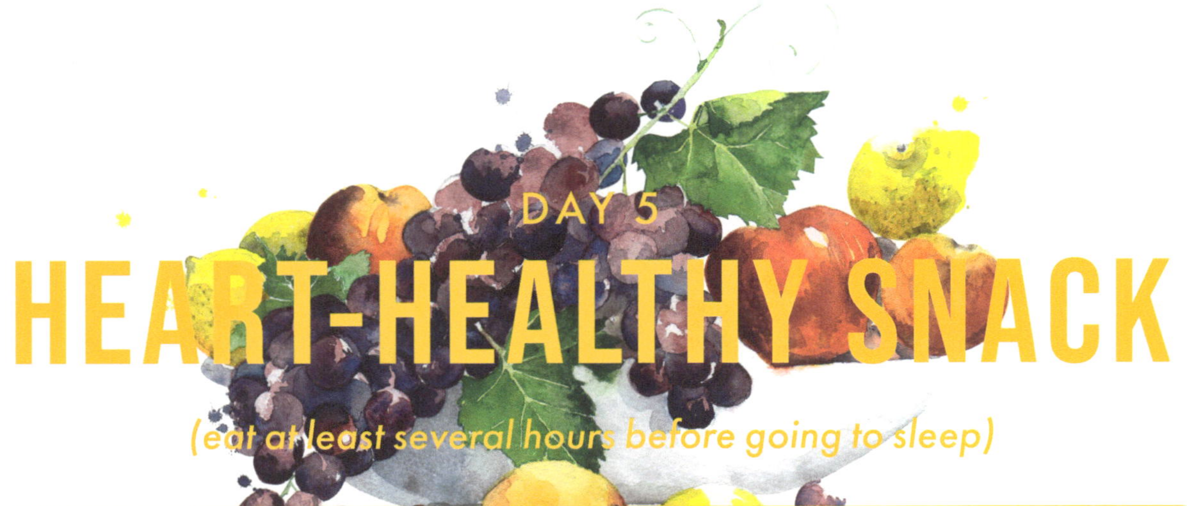

HEART-HEALTHY SNACK

(eat at least several hours before going to sleep)

- ½ cup red grapes
- ½ apple

Snack Benefits

RED GRAPES – contain a high concentration of potassium, which helps maintain proper water and electrolyte balance to sustain normal blood pressure and prevent hypertension; also contain resveratrol and vitamin C, strong antioxidants that reduce oxygen free radicals, oxidative stress, and inflammation, which prevents vascular damage and injury.

APPLE — contains a high concentration of vitamins C and B6, strong antioxidants that reduce oxygen free radicals, oxidative stress, and inflammation, which prevents vascular damage and injury; also contains magnesium and fiber, which reduces blood pressure, LDL (bad) cholesterol, blood glucose, and body weight and therefore helps prevent hypertension, atherosclerosis, diabetes, and obesity.

Snack Calculations

Snack Total	Calories	Lean Protein	Complex Carbohydrates	Unsaturated Fat	Fiber
	112	1 gm	29 gm	0 gm	3 gm

Daily Total Calculations

Daily Total	Calories	Lean Protein	Complex Carbohydrates	Unsaturated Fat	Fiber
	1854	88 gm	244 gm	72 gm	60 gm

BREAKFAST

NON-DAIRY YOGURT WITH GRANOLA AND FRESH FRUIT

- 12-ounce bowl of non-dairy yogurt (almond or oat-based)
- ½ cup classic whole grain rolled oats granola
- ½ banana
- ½ cup blueberries
- ½ apple

no added sugar or honey

Meal Benefits

NON-DIARY YOGURT – contains lean protein, which sustains healthy vascular function; contributes calcium and fiber, which reduces blood pressure, LDL (bad) cholesterol, blood glucose, and body weight and therefore helps prevent hypertension, atherosclerosis, diabetes, and obesity; provides healthy unsaturated fats, which lowers LDL (bad) cholesterol, increases HDL (good) cholesterol, and helps prevent atherosclerosis; also contains probiotics, which maintains healthy gut bacteria and intestinal health which reduces systemic inflammation that contributes to vascular damage and injury.

GRANOLA – contains a high concentration of soluble fiber, which reduces LDL (bad) cholesterol, blood glucose, blood pressure, and body weight and helps prevent atherosclerosis, diabetes, hypertension, and obesity; soluble fiber also promotes healthy gut bacteria and intestinal health which reduces systemic inflammation that contributes to vascular damage and injury; also contributes vitamin B1, manganese, and phytonutrients, potent antioxidants that reduce oxygen free radicals, oxidative stress, and inflammation, which prevents vascular damage and injury.

BANANA – contains vitamin C, an antioxidant that reduces oxygen free radicals, oxidative stress, and inflammation, which prevents vascular damage and injury; also contains a high concentration of potassium and fiber, which helps prevent hypertension, atherosclerosis, diabetes, and obesity by reducing blood pressure, LDL (bad) cholesterol, blood glucose, and body weight.

BLUEBERRIES – contain the highest concentration of the antioxidants anthocyanins among all fresh fruits, reducing oxygen free radicals, oxidative stress, and inflammation, which prevents vascular damage and injury; also contain a high concentration of vitamin C and soluble fiber, which reduces blood pressure, LDL (bad) cholesterol, blood glucose, and body weight and therefore helps prevent hypertension, atherosclerosis, diabetes, and obesity.

APPLE — contains a high concentration of vitamins C and B6, strong antioxidants that reduce oxygen free radicals, oxidative stress, and inflammation, which prevents vascular damage and injury; also contains magnesium and fiber, which reduces blood pressure, LDL (bad) cholesterol, blood glucose, and body weight and therefore helps prevent hypertension, atherosclerosis, diabetes, and obesity.

Breakfast Calculations

Meal Total	Calories	Lean Protein	Complex Carbohydrates	Unsaturated Fat	Fiber
	583	17 gm	68 gm	30 gm	21 gm

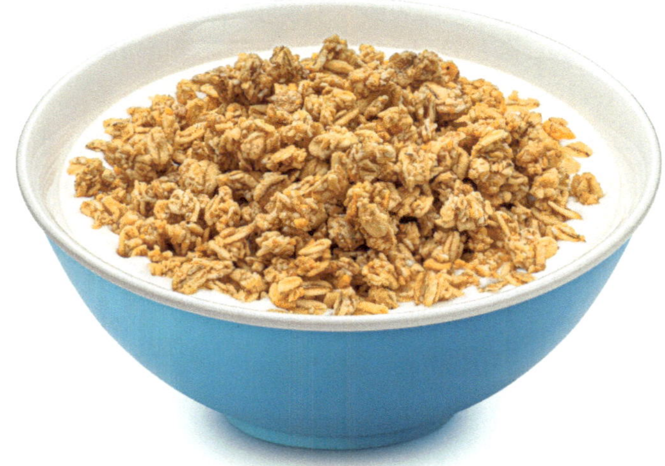

LUNCH

VEGETABLE SALAD WITH CHICKPEAS

- 2 cups kale
- 1 cup of chickpeas (*drain and rinse with cold water before eating*)
- ½ red bell pepper
- ½ cucumber
- 1 garlic clove, chopped
- ½ red onion, sliced

Olive oil vinaigrette – mix and add as salad dressing

- 2 tablespoons extra-virgin olive oil
- 1 tablespoon apple wine vinegar
- 1 teaspoon black pepper

Meal Benefits

KALE – contains vitamin C and phytonutrients, antioxidants that reduce oxygen free radicals, oxidative stress, and inflammation, which prevents vascular damage and injury; also contains vitamin D, calcium, and fiber, which reduces blood pressure, LDL (bad) cholesterol, blood glucose, and body weight and therefore helps prevent hypertension, atherosclerosis, diabetes, and obesity.

CHICKPEAS — contain lean protein, iron, and soluble fiber, which sustains healthy vascular function, prevents anemia, reduces blood pressure, LDL (bad) cholesterol, blood glucose, and body weight, and therefore helps prevent atherosclerosis, hypertension, diabetes, and obesity.

RED BELL PEPPER – contains high levels of the antioxidants vitamins C and B6 that reduce oxygen free radicals, oxidative stress, and inflammation, which prevents vascular damage and injury; also contributes potassium and soluble fiber, which reduces blood pressure, LDL (bad) cholesterol, blood

glucose, and body weight and therefore helps prevent hypertension, atherosclerosis, diabetes, and obesity.

CUCUMBER UNPEELED (PEELING REDUCES THE AMOUNT OF FIBER, VITAMINS, AND MINERALS) – contains vitamin C, a strong antioxidant that reduces oxygen free radicals, oxidative stress, and inflammation, which prevents vascular damage and injury; provides magnesium and potassium, essential minerals that help maintain proper water and electrolyte balance to sustain normal blood pressure and prevent hypertension; also provides fiber, which reduces LDL (bad) cholesterol, blood glucose, and body weight, and therefore helps prevent atherosclerosis, diabetes, and obesity.

GARLIC – contains allicin, a powerful antioxidant that reduces oxygen free radicals, oxidative stress, and inflammation, which prevents vascular damage and injury; also contains vitamin C and fiber, which reduces blood pressure, LDL (bad) cholesterol, blood glucose, and body weight and therefore helps prevent hypertension, atherosclerosis, diabetes, and obesity.

RED ONIONS – contain the powerful antioxidants quercetin and vitamin C that reduce oxygen free radicals, oxidative stress, and inflammation, which prevents vascular damage and injury; also contribute calcium and fiber, which reduces blood pressure,

LDL (bad) cholesterol, blood glucose, and body weight and therefore helps prevent hypertension, atherosclerosis, diabetes, and obesity.

OLIVE OIL – contains a high concentration of oleocanthal and vitamin E, powerful antioxidants that reduce oxygen free radicals, oxidative stress, and inflammation, which prevents vascular damage and injury; also provides a high concentration of monounsaturated fats, which lowers LDL (bad) cholesterol, increases HDL (good) cholesterol and therefore helps prevent atherosclerosis.

APPLE CIDER VINEGAR – contains polyphenols, powerful antioxidants that reduce oxygen free radicals, oxidative stress, and inflammation, which prevents vascular damage and injury; also contains acetic acid which lowers LDL (bad) cholesterol, blood pressure, blood glucose levels, and body weight and therefore helps prevent atherosclerosis, hypertension, diabetes, and obesity.

BLACK PEPPER –contains the powerful antioxidant piperine that reduces oxygen free radicals, oxidative stress, and inflammation, which prevents vascular damage and injury; also contains potassium, calcium, and magnesium, essential minerals that lower blood pressure and LDL (bad) cholesterol levels and therefore help prevent hypertension and atherosclerosis.

Lunch Calculations

Meal Total	Calories	Lean Protein	Complex Carbohydrates	Unsaturated Fat	Fiber
	529	15 gm	55 gm	31 gm	18 gm

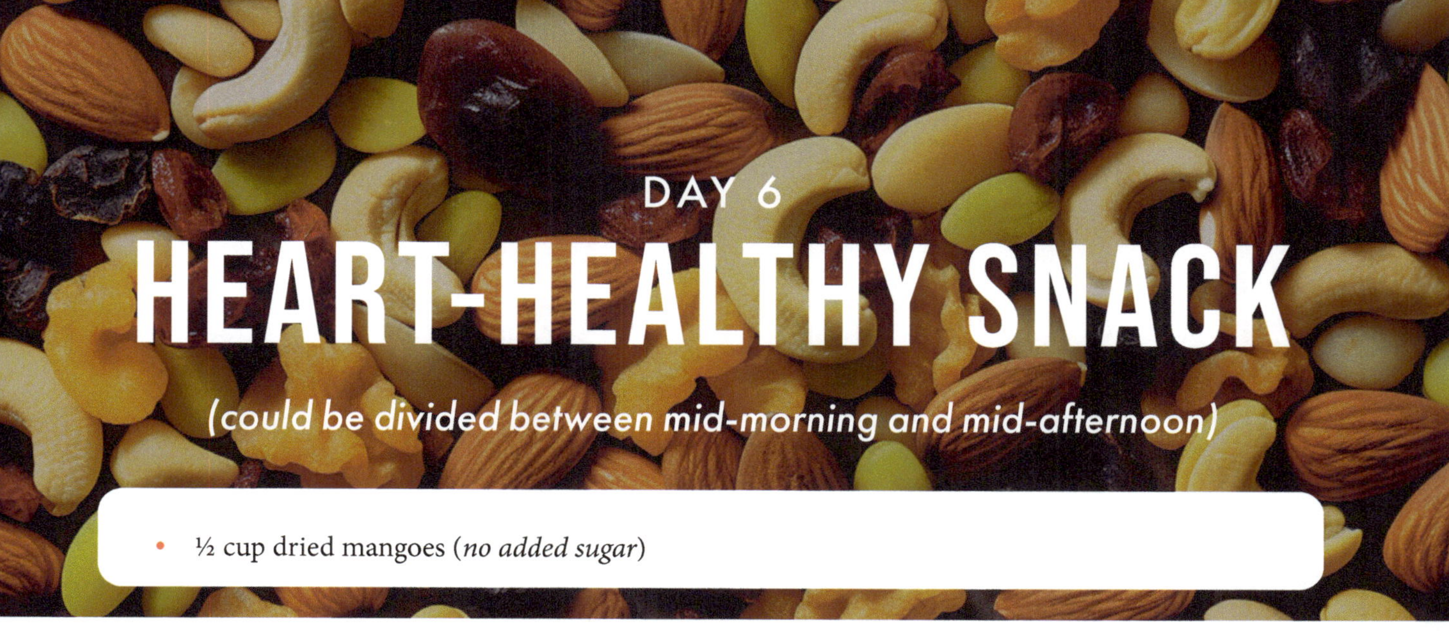

HEART-HEALTHY SNACK

(could be divided between mid-morning and mid-afternoon)

- ½ cup dried mangoes (*no added sugar*)

Snack Benefits

DRIED MANGOES – an excellent source of the potent antioxidant beta-carotene that reduces oxygen free radicals, oxidative stress, and inflammation, which prevents vascular damage and injury; also provides magnesium and potassium, essential minerals that help maintain normal blood pressure to prevent hypertension; in addition, provides an excellent source of fiber which reduces LDL (bad) cholesterol, blood glucose, blood pressure, and body weight.

Snack Calculations

Snack Total	Calories	Lean Protein	Complex Carbohydrates	Unsaturated Fat	Fiber
	160	1 gm	38 gm	0 gm	2 gm

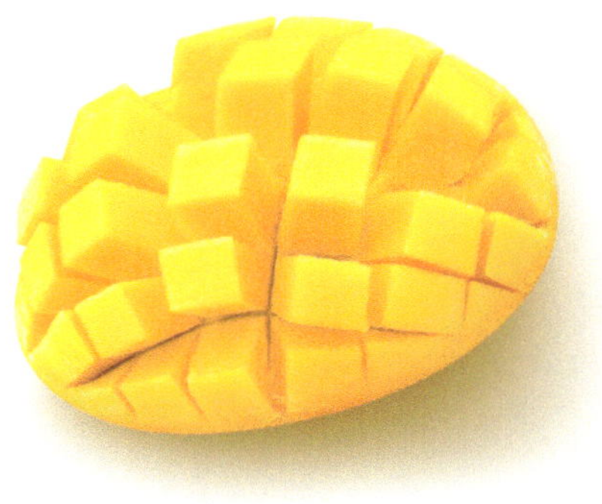

DINNER

BAKED SALMON AND VEGETABLE MIX WITH SWEET POTATO FRIES

- 6-ounce salmon
- ½ green bell pepper, sliced and sauteed with:
- ½ chopped red onion
- 1 garlic clove, chopped
- 2 teaspoons extra-virgin olive oil
- ½ sweet potato fries

Season dinner meals with your choice and preference from the powdered condiments on the shopping list – salt-free garlic and onion powder are especially healthy options. Gradually eliminate seasoning food with salt as previously described in the Healthier Food Options section.

Meal Benefits

SALMON – contains high concentrations of vitamins B6 and B12, which helps maintain healthy red blood cells, prevents anemia, and therefore reduces the risk of vascular damage and injury; also provides a high concentration of polyunsaturated fats called omega-3 fatty acids, which lowers LDL (bad) cholesterol, increases HDL (good) cholesterol and therefore helps prevent atherosclerosis.

GREEN BELL PEPPER – contains high levels of the antioxidants vitamins C and B6 that reduce oxygen free radicals, oxidative stress, and inflammation, which prevents vascular damage and injury; also contributes potassium and soluble fiber, which reduces blood pressure, LDL (bad) cholesterol, blood glucose, and body weight and therefore helps prevent hypertension, atherosclerosis, diabetes, and obesity.

RED ONIONS – contain the powerful antioxidants quercetin and vitamin C that reduce oxygen free radicals, oxidative stress, and inflammation, which prevents vascular damage and injury; also contribute calcium and fiber, which reduces blood pressure, LDL (bad) cholesterol, blood glucose, and body weight and therefore helps prevent hypertension, atherosclerosis, diabetes, and obesity.

GARLIC – contains allicin, a powerful antioxidant that reduces oxygen free radicals, oxidative stress, and inflammation, which prevents vascular damage and injury; also contains vitamin C and fiber, which reduces blood pressure, LDL (bad) cholesterol, blood glucose, and body weight and therefore helps prevent hypertension, atherosclerosis, diabetes, and obesity.

OLIVE OIL – contains a high concentration of oleocanthal and vitamin E, powerful antioxidants that reduce oxygen free radicals, oxidative stress, and inflammation, which prevents vascular damage and injury; also provides a high concentration of monounsaturated fats, which lowers LDL (bad) cholesterol, increases HDL (good) cholesterol and therefore helps prevent atherosclerosis.

SWEET POTATO – contains beta-carotene and vitamins B6 and C, antioxidants that reduce oxygen free radicals, oxidative stress, and inflammation, which prevents vascular damage and injury; provides calcium, potassium, and magnesium, essential minerals that sustain healthy vascular function and reduce blood pressure, which helps prevent hypertension; also contributes soluble fiber, which reduces LDL (bad) cholesterol, blood glucose, blood pressure, and body weight, and therefore helps prevent atherosclerosis, diabetes, hypertension, and obesity.

Dinner Calculations

Meal Total	Calories	Lean Protein	Complex Carbohydrates	Unsaturated Fat	Fiber
	532	51 gm	24 gm	25 gm	4 gm

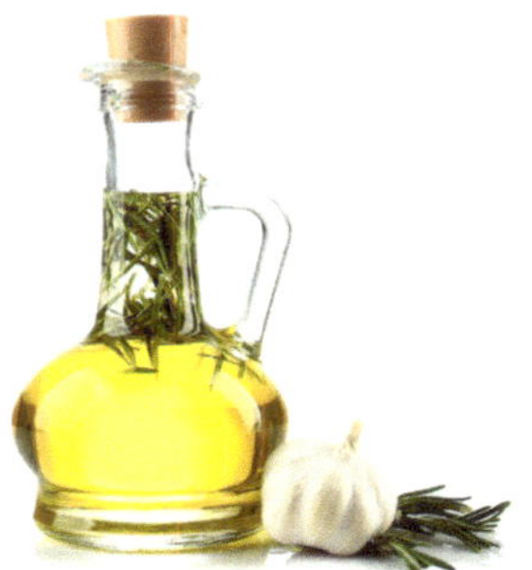

HEART-HEALTHY SNACK

(eat at least several hours before going to sleep)

- ½ cup raspberries
- ½ cup strawberries

Snack Benefits

RASPBERRIES – contain anthocyanins, antioxidants that reduce oxygen free radicals, oxidative stress, and inflammation, which prevents vascular damage and injury; also provide a high concentration of soluble fiber, potassium, and manganese which reduces LDL (bad) cholesterol, blood glucose, body weight, and blood pressure and therefore helps prevent atherosclerosis, diabetes, obesity, and hypertension.

STRAWBERRIES – contain the antioxidants vitamin C, anthocyanins, and quercetin that reduce oxygen free radicals, oxidative stress, and inflammation, which prevents vascular damage and injury; also contribute soluble fiber, which reduces LDL (bad) cholesterol, blood glucose, blood pressure, and body weight and therefore helps prevent atherosclerosis, diabetes, hypertension, and obesity.

Snack Calculations

Snack Total	Calories	Lean Protein	Complex Carbohydrates	Unsaturated Fat	Fiber
	83	1 gm	20 gm	0 gm	7 gm

Daily Total Calculations

Daily Total	Calories	Lean Protein	Complex Carbohydrates	Unsaturated Fat	Fiber
	1887	85 gm	205 gm	86 gm	52 gm

BREAKFAST

OATMEAL WITH FRESH FRUIT

- 12-ounce bowl of traditional old-fashioned oatmeal cooked with 1½ cups unsweetened, unflavored non-dairy milk (almond or oat-based)
- ½ cup raspberries
- ½ orange
- ½ cup of strawberries

no added sugar or honey

Meal Benefits

OATMEAL – contains a high concentration of the soluble fiber beta-glucan, which reduces LDL (bad) cholesterol, blood glucose, blood pressure, and body weight and therefore helps prevent atherosclerosis, diabetes, hypertension, and obesity; beta-glucan also promotes healthy gut bacteria and intestinal health which reduces systemic inflammation that contributes to vascular damage and injury; also contributes vitamin B1, manganese, and phytonutrients, potent antioxidants that reduce oxygen free radicals, oxidative stress, and inflammation, which prevents vascular damage and injury.

NON-DAIRY MILK (ALMOND OR OAT-BASED) – contains no cholesterol, and lower total calories and sugar than dairy milk, reducing the risk of atherosclerosis and diabetes; also contributes lean protein and calcium, two nutrients that help sustain healthy vascular function, regulate normal blood pressure, and prevent hypertension.

RASPBERRIES – contain anthocyanins, antioxidants that reduce oxygen free radicals, oxidative stress, and inflammation, which prevents vascular damage and injury; also provide a high concentration of soluble fiber, potassium, and manganese which reduces LDL (bad) cholesterol, blood glucose, body weight, and blood pressure and therefore helps prevent atherosclerosis, diabetes, obesity, and hypertension.

ORANGE – contains a high level of vitamin C, an antioxidant that reduces oxygen free radicals, oxidative stress, and inflammation, which prevents vascular damage and injury; also contains potassium and soluble fiber, which helps maintain proper water and electrolyte balance to reduce blood pressure, and lowers LDL (bad) cholesterol, blood glucose,

and body weight, which helps prevent hypertension, atherosclerosis, diabetes, and obesity.

STRAWBERRIES – contain the antioxidants vitamin C, anthocyanins, and quercetin that reduce oxygen free radicals, oxidative stress, and inflammation, which prevents vascular damage and injury; also contribute soluble fiber, which reduces LDL (bad) cholesterol, blood glucose, blood pressure, and body weight and therefore helps prevent atherosclerosis, diabetes, hypertension, and obesity.

Breakfast Calculations

Meal Total	Calories	Lean Protein	Complex Carbohydrates	Unsaturated Fat	Fiber
	514	17 gm	100 gm	9 gm	18 gm

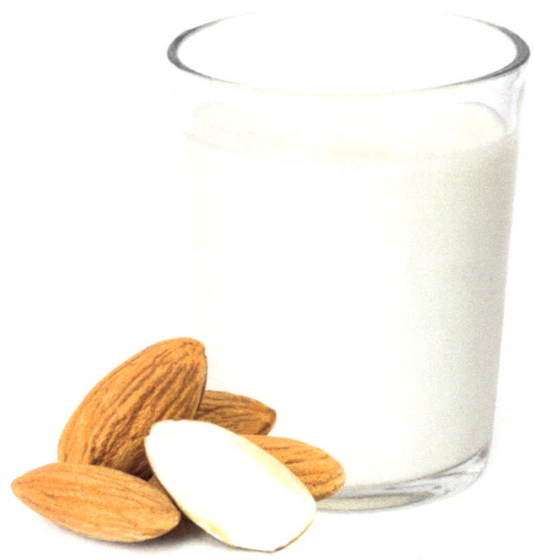

LUNCH

VEGETABLE SALAD WITH KIDNEY BEANS

- 2 cups baby spinach
- 1 cup kidney beans (*drain and rinse with cold water before eating*)
- ½ cup tomatoes
- ½ avocado
- ½ cup carrots
- ½ cup uncooked broccoli

Olive oil vinaigrette – mix and add as salad dressing

- 2 tablespoons extra-virgin olive oil
- 1 tablespoon apple wine vinegar
- 1 teaspoon oregano

Meal Benefits

SPINACH – contains phytonutrients and vitamin C, potent antioxidants that reduce oxygen free radicals, oxidative stress, and inflammation, which prevents vascular damage and injury; also contributes vitamin D, calcium, and fiber, which reduces blood pressure, LDL (bad) cholesterol, blood glucose, and body weight and therefore helps prevent hypertension, atherosclerosis, diabetes, and obesity.

KIDNEY BEANS — contain lean protein, iron, and soluble fiber, which sustains healthy vascular function, prevents anemia, reduces blood pressure, LDL (bad) cholesterol, blood glucose, and body weight, and therefore helps prevent hypertension, atherosclerosis, diabetes, and obesity.

TOMATOES – contain lycopene and vitamins B, C, and E, powerful antioxidants that reduce oxygen free radicals, oxidative stress, and inflammation, which prevents vascular damage and injury; also contain a high concentration of potassium, which lowers blood pressure to prevent hypertension.

AVOCADO – contains healthy monounsaturated fats, which lowers LDL (bad) cholesterol, increases HDL (good) cholesterol, and therefore helps prevent atherosclerosis; contributes the antioxidants vitamins C and E, and copper that reduce oxygen free radicals, oxidative stress, and inflammation, which prevents vascular damage and injury; also provides manganese which reduces blood pressure and therefore helps prevent hypertension.

CARROTS – contain vitamins A and C, and beta-carotene, strong antioxidants that reduce oxygen free radicals, oxidative stress, and inflammation, which prevents vascular damage and injury; also contribute fiber, which reduces LDL (bad) cholesterol, blood glucose, blood pressure, and body weight and therefore helps prevent atherosclerosis, diabetes, hypertension, and obesity.

BROCCOLI – contains flavonoids, carotenoids including lutein and beta-carotene, and vitamin C, which are powerful antioxidants that reduce oxygen free radicals, oxidative stress, and inflammation, which prevents vascular damage and injury; also contains a high concentration of soluble fiber, which reduces LDL (bad) cholesterol, blood glucose, blood pressure, and body weight, and therefore helps prevent atherosclerosis, diabetes, hypertension, and obesity.

OLIVE OIL – contains a high concentration of oleocanthal and vitamin E, powerful antioxidants that reduce oxygen free radicals, oxidative stress, and inflammation, which prevents vascular damage and injury; also provides a high concentration of monounsaturated fats, which lowers LDL (bad) cholesterol, increases HDL (good) cholesterol and therefore helps prevent atherosclerosis.

RED WINE VINEGAR – contains polyphenols, powerful antioxidants that reduce oxygen free radicals, oxidative stress, and inflammation, which prevents vascular damage and injury; also contains acetic acid which lowers LDL (bad) cholesterol, blood pressure, blood glucose levels, and body weight and therefore helps prevent atherosclerosis, hypertension, diabetes, and obesity.

OREGANO – contains a high concentration of polyphenol antioxidants, including carvacrol, that reduce oxygen free radicals, oxidative stress, and inflammation, which prevents vascular damage and injury; also provides high levels of calcium, which is essential to normal cardiac and vascular function and helps reduce blood pressure and therefore prevent hypertension.

Lunch Calculations

Meal Total	Calories	Lean Protein	Complex Carbohydrates	Unsaturated Fat	Fiber
	539	13 gm	40 gm	39 gm	17 gm

HEART-HEALTHY SNACK

(could be divided between mid-morning and mid-afternoon)

- ½ cup of walnuts (*raw, no added salt or sugar/honey*)

Snack Benefits

WALNUTS: an excellent source of copper, an antioxidant mineral that reduces oxygen free radicals, oxidative stress, and inflammation, which prevents vascular damage and injury; also contribute manganese and magnesium, essential minerals that reduce blood pressure and LDL (bad) cholesterol; in addition, contain high levels of lean protein, unsaturated fats, and soluble fiber, which sustains healthy vascular function and reduces LDL (bad) cholesterol, blood glucose, and body weight.

Snack Calculations

Snack Total	Calories	Lean Protein	Complex Carbohydrates	Unsaturated Fat	Fiber
	392	9 gm	8 gm	39 gm	3 gm

DINNER

SAUTEED COD LOIN FILET AND RED CABBAGE WITH SWEET POTATO

- 6-ounce cod loin filet
- sauteed red cabbage with 2 teaspoons extra-virgin olive oil:
- 1 cup raw red cabbage, shredded
- 1 teaspoon paprika
- ½ teaspoon oregano
- 1 garlic clove, minced
- 1 sliced sweet potato, sauteed or baked

Season dinner meals with your choice and preference from the powdered condiments on the shopping list – salt-free garlic and onion powder are especially healthy options. Gradually eliminate seasoning food with salt as previously described in the Healthier Food Options section.

Meal Benefits

COD – contains lean protein and high concentrations of vitamins B6 and B12, which helps maintain healthy vascular function, prevents anemia, and therefore reduces the risk of vascular damage and injury; provides a high concentration of polyunsaturated fats called omega-3 fatty acids, which lowers LDL (bad) cholesterol, increases HDL (good) cholesterol and therefore helps prevent atherosclerosis; also contributes phosphorus, an antioxidant that reduces oxygen free radicals, oxidative stress, and inflammation, which prevents vascular damage and injury.

RED CABBAGE – contains vitamin C, a strong antioxidant that reduces oxygen free radicals, oxidative stress, and inflammation, which prevents vascular damage and injury; also provides soluble fiber that reduces LDL (bad) cholesterol, blood glucose, blood pressure, and body weight, and therefore helps prevent atherosclerosis, diabetes hypertension, and obesity.

PAPRIKA –contains carotenoids and vitamins A, B6, C, and E, all powerful antioxidants that reduce oxygen free radicals, oxidative stress, and inflammation, which prevents vascular damage and injury; also provides potassium, which lowers blood pressure and therefore helps prevent hypertension.

OREGANO – contains a high concentration of polyphenol antioxidants, including carvacrol, that reduce oxygen free radicals, oxidative stress, and inflammation, which prevents vascular damage and injury; also provides high levels of calcium, which is essential to normal cardiac and vascular function and helps reduce blood pressure and therefore prevent hypertension.

GARLIC – contains allicin, a powerful antioxidant that reduces oxygen free radicals, oxidative stress, and inflammation, which prevents vascular damage and injury; also contains vitamin C and fiber, which reduces blood pressure, LDL (bad) cholesterol, blood

glucose, and body weight and therefore helps prevent hypertension, atherosclerosis, diabetes, and obesity.

SWEET POTATO – contains beta-carotene and vitamins B6 and C, antioxidants that reduce oxygen free radicals, oxidative stress, and inflammation, which prevents vascular damage and injury; provides calcium, potassium, and magnesium, essential minerals that sustain healthy vascular function and reduce blood pressure, which helps prevent hypertension; also contributes soluble fiber, which reduces LDL (bad) cholesterol, blood glucose, blood pressure, and body weight, and therefore helps prevent atherosclerosis, diabetes, hypertension, and obesity.

OLIVE OIL – contains a high concentration of oleocanthal and vitamin E, powerful antioxidants that reduce oxygen free radicals, oxidative stress, and inflammation, which prevents vascular damage and injury; also provides a high concentration of monounsaturated fats, which lowers LDL (bad) cholesterol, increases HDL (good) cholesterol and therefore helps prevent atherosclerosis.

Dinner Calculations

Meal Total	Calories	Lean Protein	Complex Carbohydrates	Unsaturated Fat	Fiber
	472	44 gm	29 gm	19 gm	6 gm

HEART-HEALTHY SNACK

(eat at least several hours before going to sleep)

- ½ cup red grapes
- ½ cup blueberries

Snack Benefits

RED GRAPES – contain a high concentration of potassium, which helps maintain proper water and electrolyte balance to sustain normal blood pressure and prevent hypertension; also contain resveratrol and vitamin C, strong antioxidants that reduce oxygen free radicals, oxidative stress, and inflammation, which prevents vascular damage and injury.

BLUEBERRIES – contain the highest concentration of the antioxidants anthocyanins among all fresh fruits, reducing oxygen free radicals, oxidative stress, and inflammation, which prevents vascular damage and injury; also contain a high concentration of vitamin C and soluble fiber, which reduces blood pressure, LDL (bad) cholesterol, blood glucose, and body weight and therefore helps prevent hypertension, atherosclerosis, diabetes, and obesity.

Snack Calculations

Snack Total	Calories	Lean Protein	Complex Carbohydrates	Unsaturated Fat	Fiber
	100	2 gm	25 gm	0 gm	3 gm

Daily Total Calculations

Daily Total	Calories	Lean Protein	Complex Carbohydrates	Unsaturated Fat	Fiber
	2017	85 gm	202 gm	106 gm	47 gm

DAILY AVERAGE TOTAL CALCULATIONS FOR 21-MEAL PLAN

Daily Average	Calories	Lean Protein	Complex Carbohydrates	Unsaturated Fat	Fiber
	1892	85 gm	225 gm	82 gm	51 gm

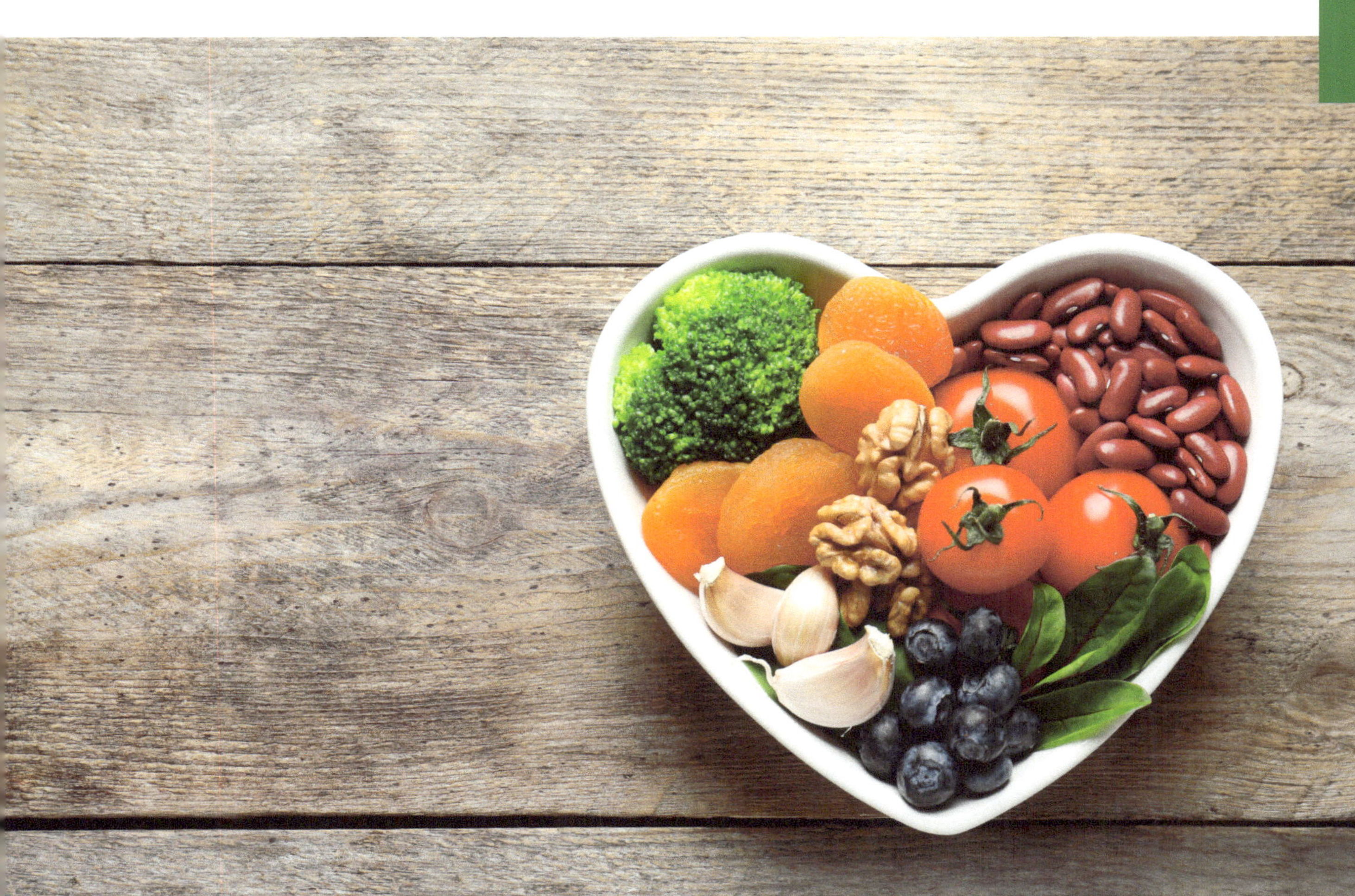

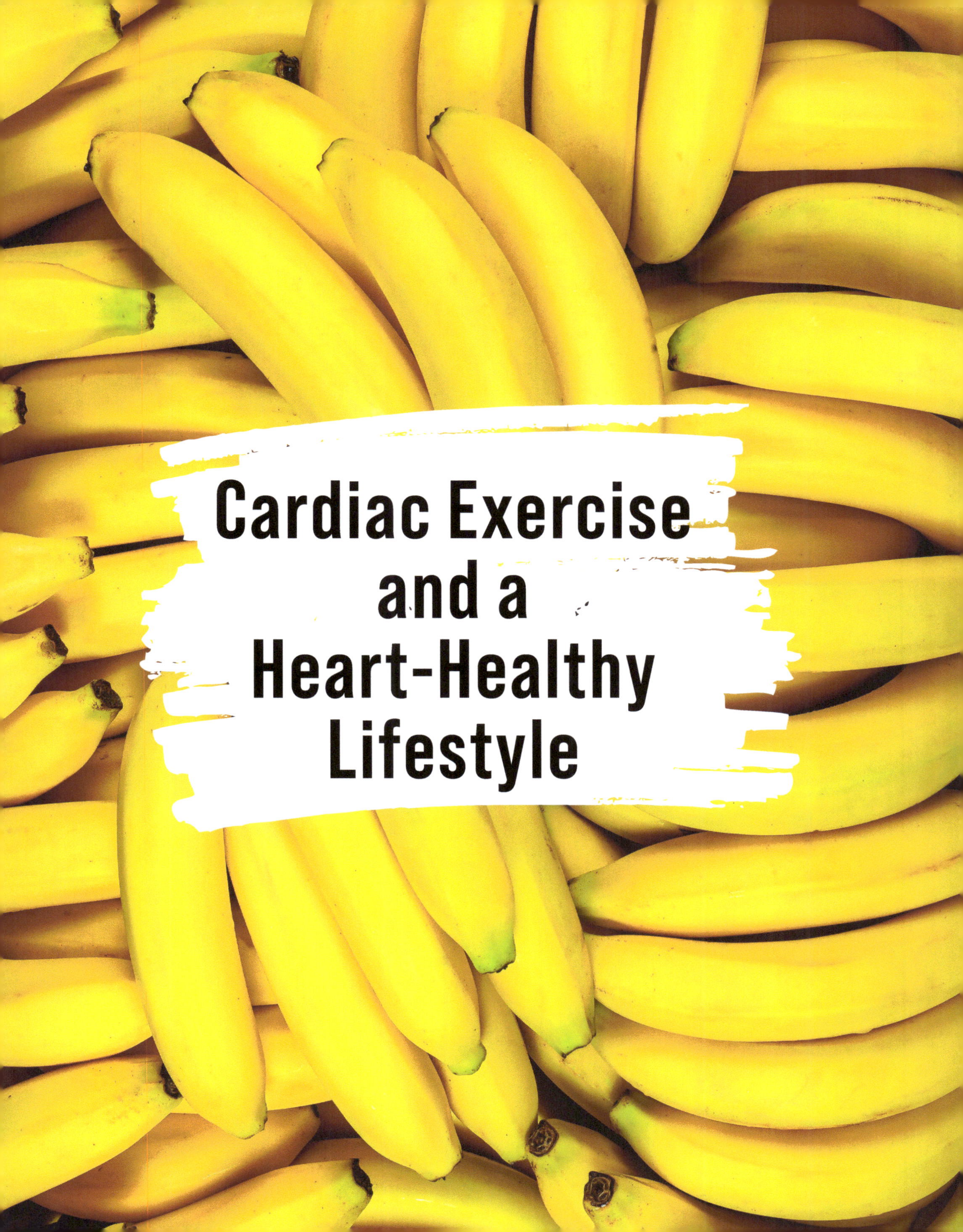
Cardiac Exercise
and a
Heart-Healthy
Lifestyle

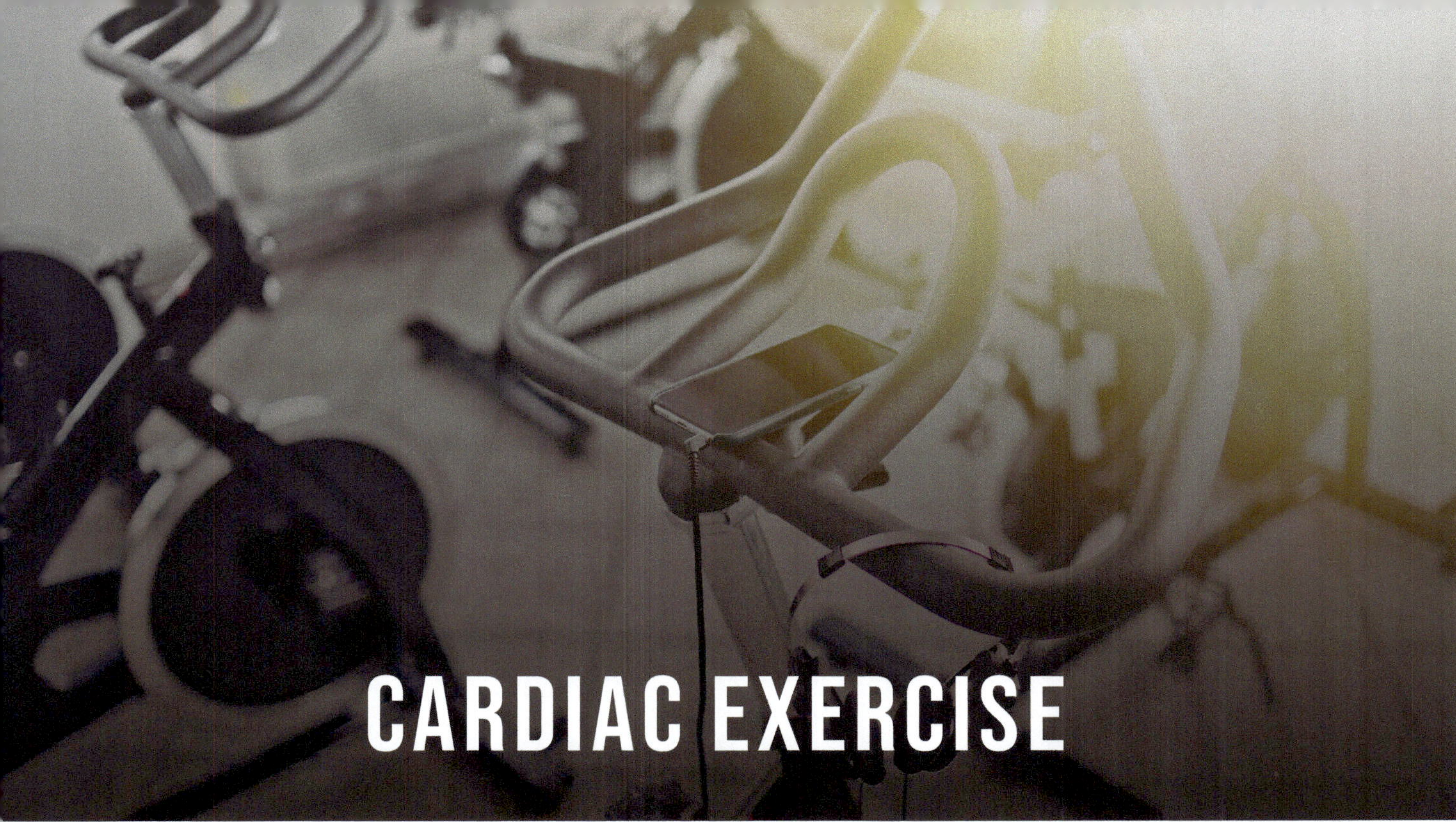

CARDIAC EXERCISE

Cardiac exercise (aerobic, cardio) involves physical activities that elevate the heart rate for an extended time. This primarily includes fast-paced walking, jogging, and cycling and is an essential evidence-based health-promoting behavior.

Basic science studies have revealed that the body's biochemical response to cardiac exercise promotes antioxidant activity, which reduces systemic inflammation, oxygen free radicals, and oxidative stress, and therefore prevents vascular damage and injury. Clinical studies have demonstrated that regular cardiac exercise significantly decreases the risk of cardiovascular diseases, increases longevity, improves blood pressure, blood cholesterol, and blood glucose, and also lowers body weight and alleviates stress.

Underserved communities face obstacles in implementing cardiac exercise into their Health Empowerment strategy because limited financial resources often preclude purchasing gym memberships or home exercise equipment. In addition, environmental injustices result in an extreme lack of open public spaces for outdoor exercising, including free and safe access to running tracks and bicycle lanes.

Despite these challenges, incorporating regular cardiac exercise into your health-promoting routine is of vital importance, as this behavior helps you live longer and live better. Fortunately, research has revealed that fast-paced walking for 30 minutes a day, as many days a week as possible (ideally seven), is a sufficient cardiac exercise to prevent cardiovascular diseases and improve risk factors.

Using this information, patients have described in detail the benefits of forming small, community-based walking groups with family and/or friends and scheduling designated times for 30-minute fast-paced walking in their respective neighborhoods. This is an optimal cardiac exercise strategy that effectively incorporates an evidence-based health-promoting behavior, involves no financial expenditure, and promotes a community-based social activity.

This innovative and creative Health Empowerment exercise strategy reflects the ability of underserved communities to independently promote our wellness despite the challenges imposed by a healthcare system in crisis. When exercising in a gym or at home using a treadmill or stationary bicycle equipment is not possible, 30 minutes of fast-paced walking in groups in your community is enough physical activity to make everyone live longer and live better. If you are not currently exercising, gradually introduce a regular cardiac exercise regimen into your Health Empowerment strategy by starting one day a week for the first week, then adding an additional day of cardiac exercise every two weeks until you are exercising every day.

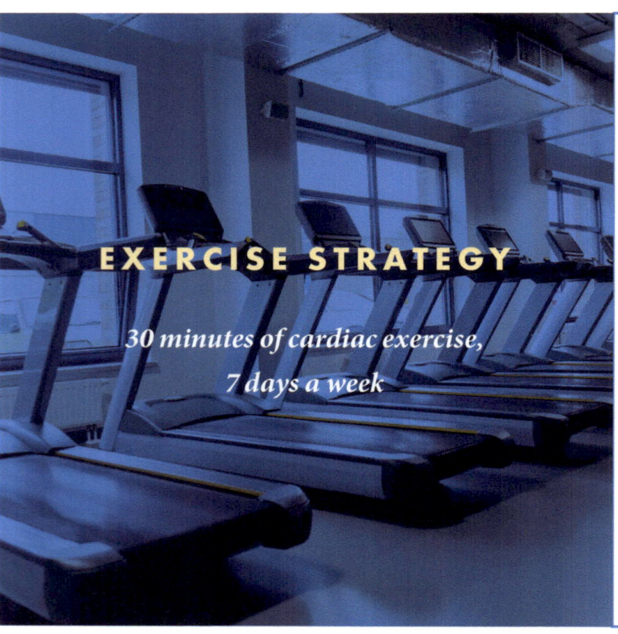

- **JOGGING** – gym treadmill, home treadmill, community track if accessible
- **CYCLING** – gym stationary bicycle, home stationary bicycle, community bicycle lanes if accessible and safe (always wear protective gear including helmets)
- **FAST-PACE WALKING** – gym treadmill, home treadmill, community track if accessible
- **FAST-PACE WALKING** – in your community with a walking group of family and/or friends

GRADUAL PACE FOR INTRODUCING CARDIAC EXERCISE

Initiating a cardiac exercise regimen can be challenging, to ensure consistency over time consider this gradual pace transition to incorporate regular physical activity into your Health Empowerment strategy:

Select one day of the week to exercise for the first week, then introduce an additional day every two weeks while always exercising on the days you already started. Start on the most convenient day for you based on available time in your schedule.

Example:

WEEK ONE: Start 30 minutes of cardiac exercise on Saturday

WEEK THREE: Continue 30 minutes of cardiac exercise every SaturdayStart 30 minutes of cardiac exercise on Sunday

WEEK FIVE: Continue 30 minutes of cardiac exercise every SaturdayContinue 30 minutes of cardiac exercise every SundayStart 30 minutes of cardiac exercise on Monday

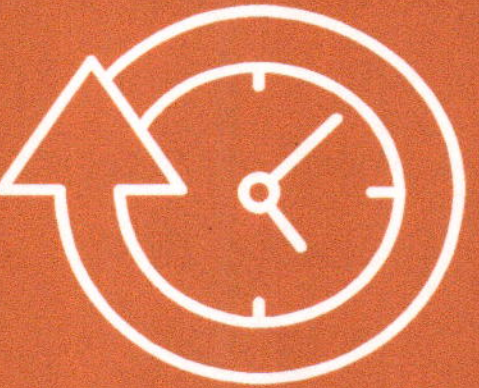

Continue this pattern for 14 weeks (approximately 3.5 months) until you have incorporated 30 minutes of cardiac exercise, 7 days a week.

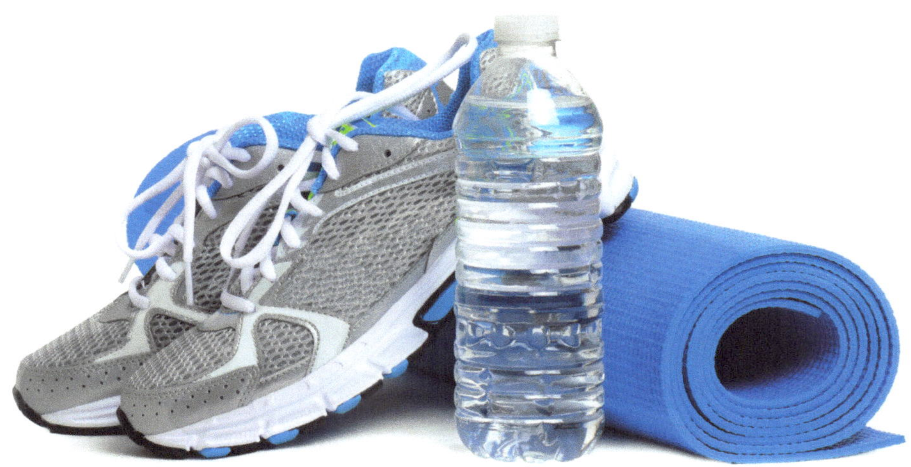

NICOTINE DEPENDENCE

Nicotine is a harmful chemical that accelerates the vascular damage and injury caused by oxygen free radicals, oxidative stress, and systemic inflammation. It significantly increases the progression of atherosclerosis and the risk of cardiovascular diseases, in addition to causing many cancers.

Nicotine dependence, in the form of cigarette smoking, vaping, or chewing tobacco, is both the most modifiable and preventable cardiovascular risk factor and one of the most challenging to manage. Nicotine and the other chemicals in tobacco products are extremely biologically addictive. Because nicotine changes our biochemistry, it creates a physical dependence, so that when a person attempts to quit smoking, they experience severe withdrawal symptoms. Smoking, as a behavior, is also psychologically addictive. Studies have demonstrated that many tobacco users have underlying anxiety that is both worsened and relieved by nicotine, resulting in a vicious cycle of dependence.

Adding to the dangers of smoking is the fact that corporations target underserved communities with advertisements and marketing of nicotine products designed to attract new young users, representing another mechanism of exploitative societal injustice and health inequity. These companies are directly increasing the prevalence of cardiovascular diseases in underserved communities and profiting from the disparities in morbidity and mortality they create. Eliminating your use of nicotine products diminishes their ability to spread death and disease in our communities.

As challenging as it is to quit smoking or using nicotine products, it is an extremely important health behavior intervention given the proven increased risk of cardiovascular diseases and the recognized causative link to lung and many other cancers.

Fortunately, most local and state health departments have free smoking cessation programs including counseling and nicotine replacement products (nicotine patches, gum, lozenges). You can find these programs online by using the search term, "free smoking cessation program" and take advantage of the services to quit nicotine as soon as possible.

Patients who have successfully stopped using nicotine products state that the best strategy involves setting a quit date in the near future (3 to 4 months) that has personal significance, like a child's birthday, a wedding anniversary, or an important holiday. Once they have committed to that date, they slowly taper down their usage. This generally means eliminating at least one daily nicotine use each week until the quit date. When coupled with nicotine replacement aids like patches, gum, or lozenges, this reduces the concentration of nicotine in the body over time and lessens the severity of withdrawal and the probability of relapse.

For example, each week you would quit the use of a single cigarette, vape, or chew associated with a specific activity, then never use nicotine at that time again. If you always smoke a cigarette right before going to sleep, quit just that cigarette for the first week — and never use nicotine at that time again.

The next week quit another cigarette associated with an activity, such as after dinner, and continue this pattern until the quit date. Eliminating usage in stages helps improve your chances that you will completely stop on your quit date.

The cardiovascular risks associated with nicotine dependence cannot be overstated and the benefits of cessation start minutes after your last nicotine use!

NICOTINE CESSATION STRATEGY

1. Research local Department of Health "free smoking cessation program" resources online and use them as directed, including counseling and nicotine replacement products.

2. Pick a quit date in the near future (3 to 4 months) that has personal significance.

3. Quit one nicotine use a week and never smoke, vape, or chew at that time again.

EXAMPLE:

WEEK ONE: quit nicotine use before going to sleep — never use nicotine before going to sleep again

WEEK TWO: quit nicotine use after eating breakfast — never use nicotine after eating breakfast or before going to sleep again

WEEK THREE: quit nicotine use after eating lunch — never use nicotine after eating lunch, after eating breakfast, or before going to sleep ever again

Continue this pattern until your quit date and use nicotine replacement products as directed to reduce withdrawal symptoms

4. STOP using nicotine altogether on your designated quit date.

STRESS

Stress is clinically defined as external realities we experience as personal physical, mental, or emotional challenges that cause biochemical changes in our body that adversely affect our health. It is both a quantitative and qualitative cardiovascular risk factor associated with significantly increased morbidity and mortality, meaning that the risk is measurable but also individualized to the unique reality of each patient. Therefore, there is no universal strategy to eliminate stress.

The historical and current economic, political, social, and environmental injustices experienced by underserved communities increase the severity of stress (allostatic load) and its negative effect on cardiovascular health, while also limiting our resources to resolve it. Scientific studies have consistently revealed that the objective measures of stress (adrenaline and cortisol levels determined by laboratory blood tests) are significantly higher in patients from underserved communities and directly linked to increased rates of hypertension, diabetes, dyslipidemia, atherosclerosis, and death from cardiovascular diseases. The external realities that accelerate stress in underserved communities are entrenched societal injustices, including structural racism and generational poverty, which means resolving stress individually is extremely challenging.

This is why our personal journeys toward optimal health must always be linked to the struggle and movement for social justice and health equity.

Clinical studies have revealed that a heart-healthy diet and regular exercise reduce stress, so implementing the Health Empowerment strategy is the most important first step.

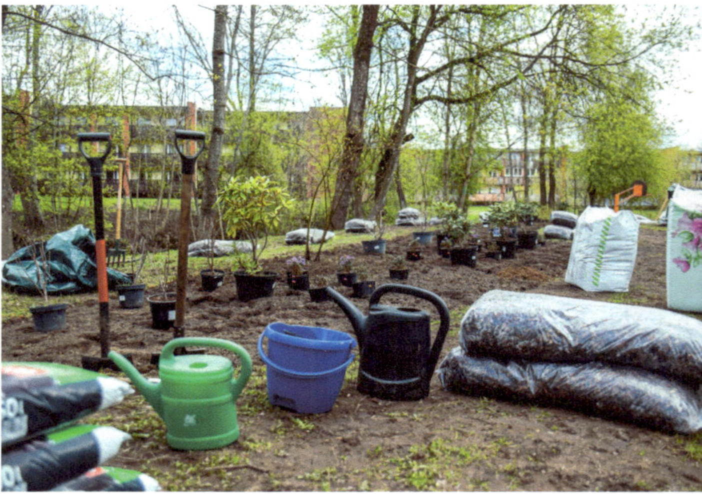

Social isolation increases stress so maximizing the time spent with family and friends is extremely important. Volunteer work is also a recognized way to engage with others and reduce stress, including informal participation. Patients with religious faith report significantly reduced stress when they increase the time they spend in spiritual fellowship and congregation with other believers.

Another important component to reducing stress is obtaining sufficient hours of restful sleep, generally defined as a minimum of 7-8 hours a day. Inadequate sleep is associated with heightened feelings of stress and an increased risk of cardiovascular diseases. But similar to stress, insomnia is a challenging area to address because the reasons for it tend to be individualized. Prioritize securing enough restful sleep and seek medical advice if insomnia persists as there may be clinical concerns associated with this condition.

Feelings of stress that limit your ability to engage in social activities can be a sign of mental health concerns and should be discussed in detail with a primary care provider.

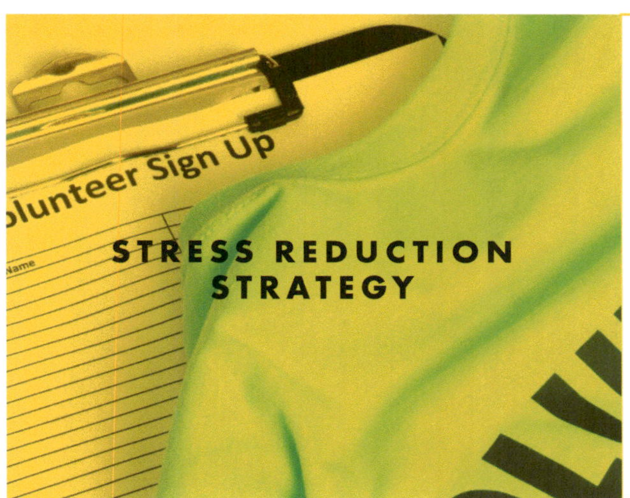

1. Health Empowerment strategy – heart-healthy diet and regular exercise
2. Maximize social time with family and friends
3. Volunteer work
4. Increase time in spiritual fellowship and congregation
5. Adequate, restful sleep 7-8 hours nightly

VITAMINS AND SUPPLEMENTS

Clinical research studies have never demonstrated a definitive association between the use of over-the-counter vitamins, minerals, antioxidants, or supplements and improved cardiovascular health. In addition, these products are often expensive, can be poorly manufactured, and may have drug interactions with prescribed medications that can be dangerous. Other than vitamins or minerals prescribed by a healthcare provider to address biological deficiencies, like vitamin B12, iron, and vitamin D, supplements have no evidence-based role in promoting wellness or reducing the risk of cardiovascular diseases. **Our resources are much better spent on fresh fruits and vegetables, that have natural vitamins, minerals, and antioxidants that definitely promote wellness.**

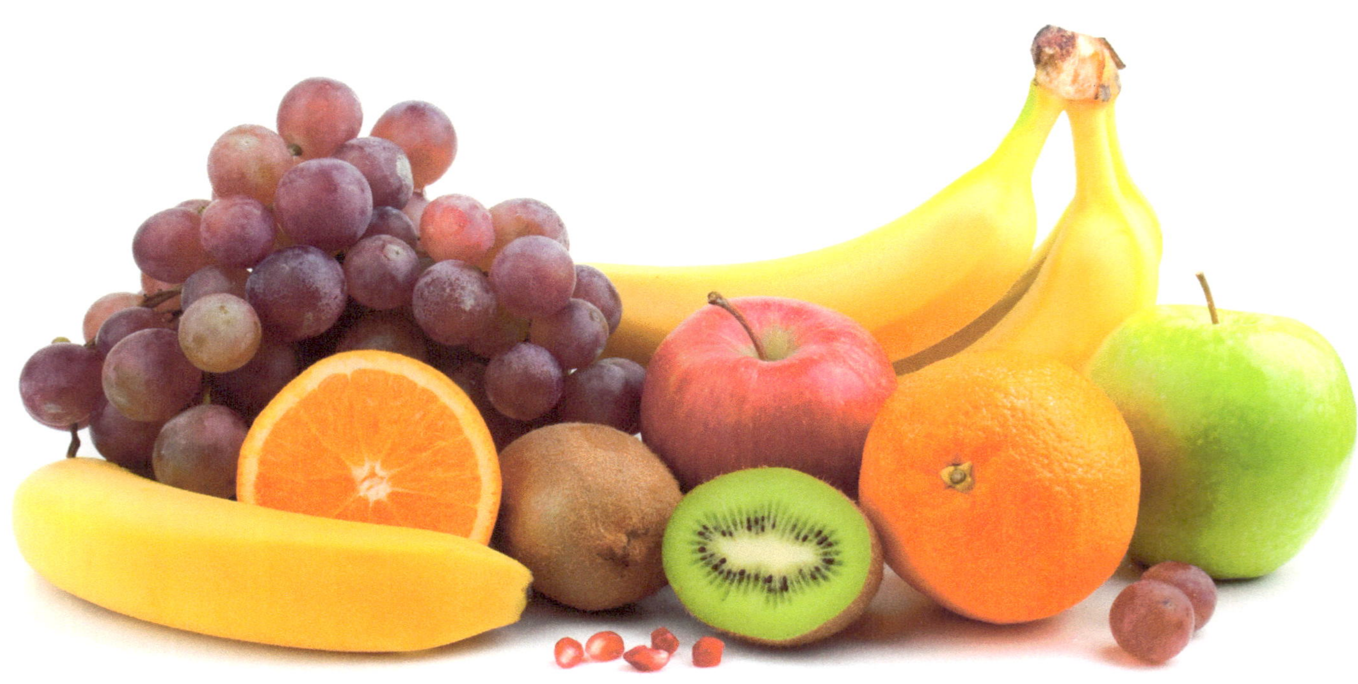

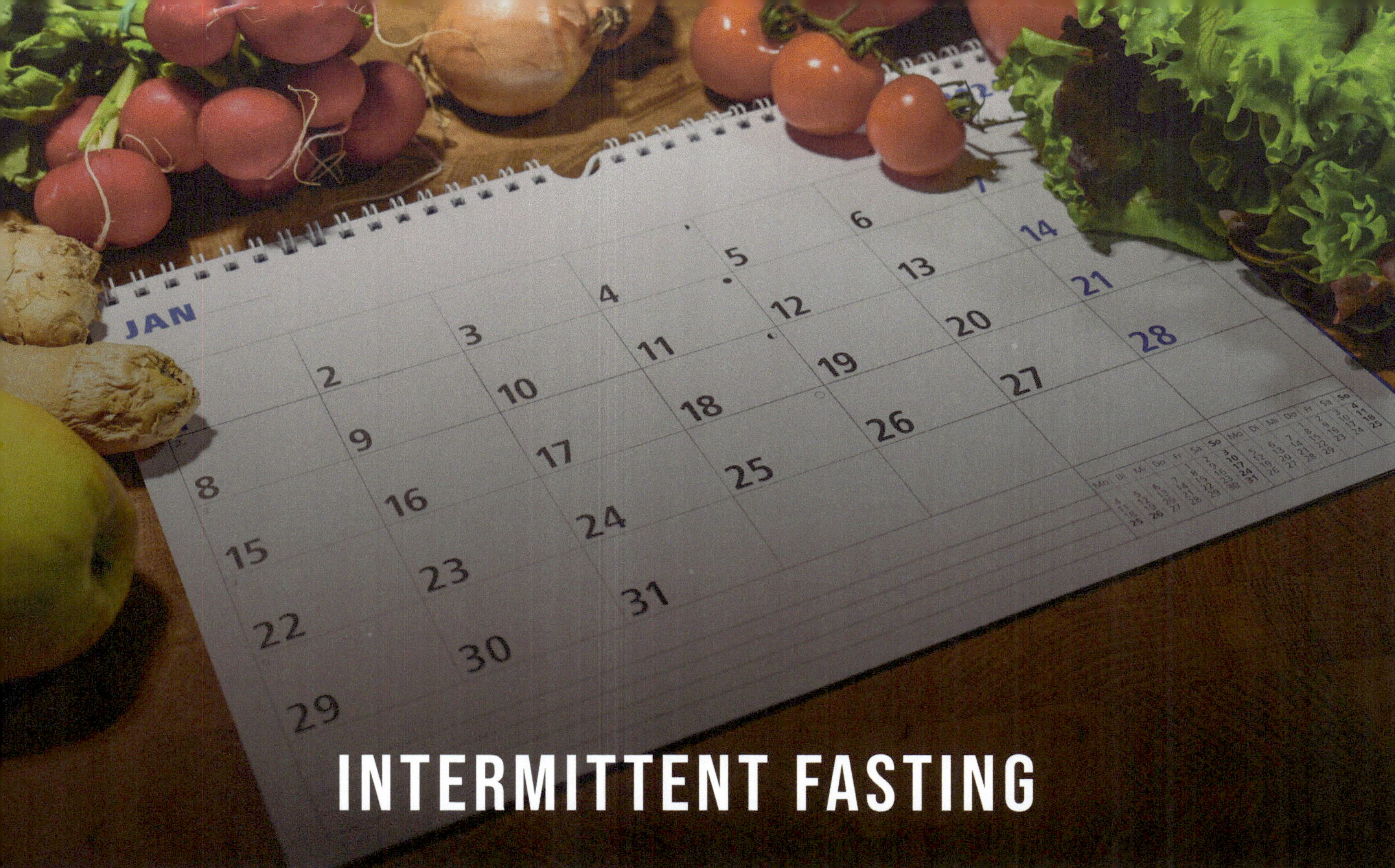

INTERMITTENT FASTING

Basic science and clinical research studies have revealed that when combined with a heart-healthy dietary plan and structured physical activity, intermittent fasting — not eating meals for a specific time period — can be a heart-healthy nutritional strategy that promotes wellness, prevents cardiovascular diseases, and helps us live longer and live better. Limiting our caloric intake by restricting when we eat has been demonstrated to reduce oxygen free radicals and oxidative stress, lower LDL (bad) cholesterol and blood glucose, improve blood pressure and HDL (good) cholesterol, and decrease body weight.

These physiological changes not only significantly reduce the risk of cardiovascular diseases but also decrease the incidence of certain cancers, help prevent dementia, and slow the progression of inflammatory diseases including asthma and arthritis. **Intermittent fasting can be part of a Health Empowerment strategy but must be done consistently and carefully. Patients with a diagnosis of diabetes requiring oral medication or insulin injections should not engage in intermittent fasting.**

There are two recognized and recommended strategies that have been determined effective when implemented over an extended time. The first is daily intermittent fasting with a **16:8 schedule**, which means eating all your meals only during an 8-hour period during the day, and only drinking water or sugar-free beverages for the remaining 16 hours of the day. For example, this could involve eating breakfast at 9 am, lunch at 1 pm, and dinner at 5 pm, and healthy snacks in between meals as necessary, but no further food consumption after 5 pm. The specific timing of each meal can vary depending on your unique schedule, but the general concept is to choose a relatively early time in the day after which you will not eat. "No food after 7 p.m." is a variation of this intermittent fasting strategy.

The other effective intermittent fasting model is the **5:2 schedule,** which involves choosing two days in the week when you only eat one meal (for example eating only an early dinner every Monday and Thursday) and eating a normal Health Empowerment meal schedule the other 5 days. This technique should be implemented gradually starting with a 6:1 schedule for one month (for example eating only an early dinner every Monday) and then proceeding to the 5:2 schedule. During the fasting days, you should remain well hydrated by drinking at least eight to ten cups (½ gallon, 2 liters) of water or sugar-free beverages throughout the day.

Intermittent fasting and caloric restriction strategies are not for everyone, involve a challenging transition period while your body and mind adapt to a new way of eating, and must be done consistently to have positive impacts on your health. However, when combined with a heart-healthy diet and regular cardiac exercise, intermittent fasting can be an essential aspect of a Health Empowerment strategy that helps underserved communities live longer and live better.

AN INTERMITTENT FASTING STRATEGY SHOULD ONLY BE IMPLEMENTED AS A HEALTH-PROMOTING BEHAVIOR, NEVER FOR FINANCIAL CONCERNS RELATED TO FOOD INSECURITY.

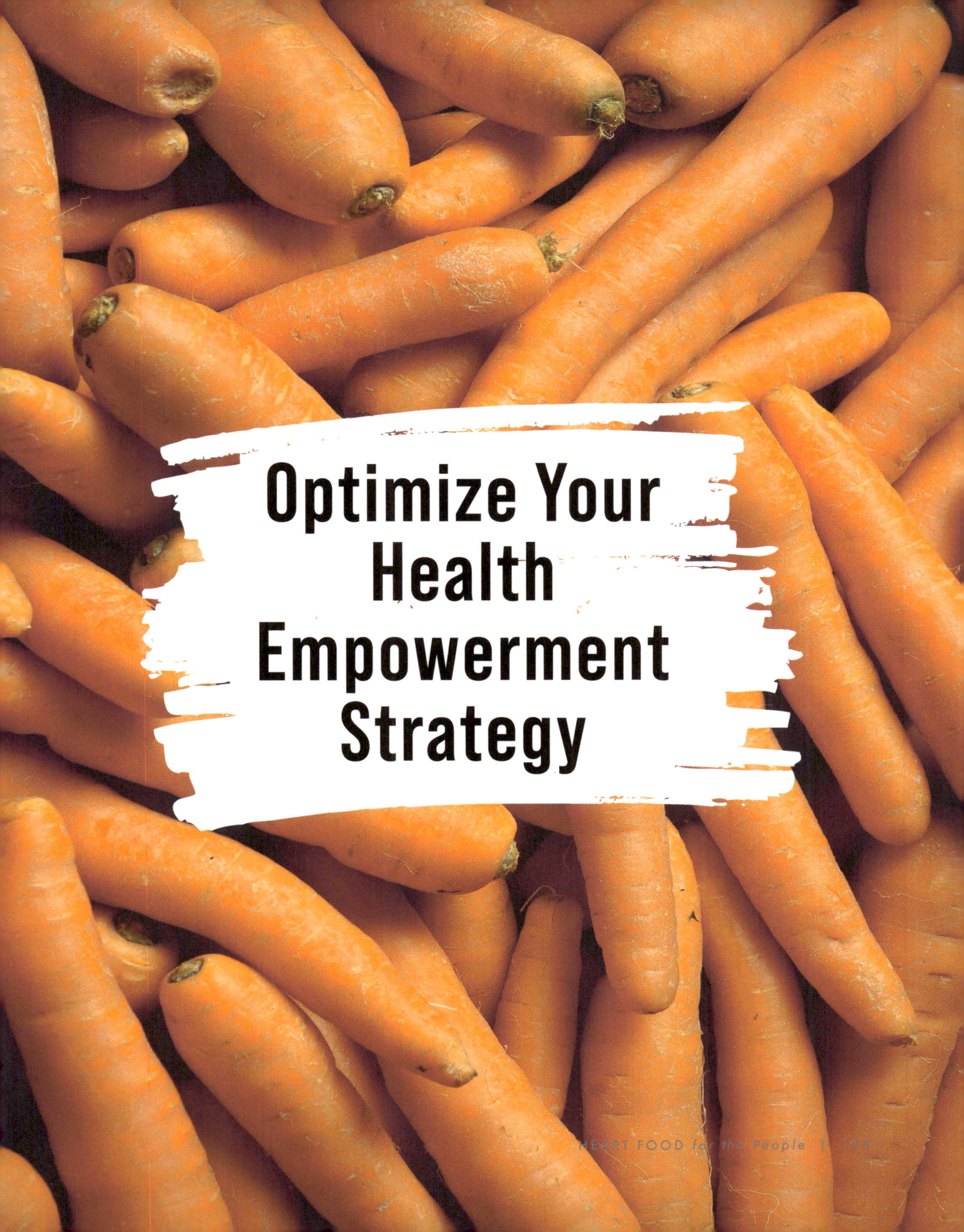

Optimize Your
Health
Empowerment
Strategy

OPTIMIZE YOUR HEALTH EMPOWERMENT STRATEGY

Given the inherent inequities and injustices of our healthcare system, the ultimate goal of Health Empowerment for underserved communities is to independently promote wellness and prevent cardiovascular diseases by implementing self-directed health-promoting behaviors and strategies.

Verifying that your strategy is working will involve some input from your healthcare providers. It is critically important that you monitor the potential risk factors that contribute to cardiovascular diseases: blood pressure, blood glucose, blood cholesterol, body weight, and nicotine use. With the support of your healthcare provider, you can optimize your Health Empowerment strategy by monitoring your cardiovascular disease risk factors.

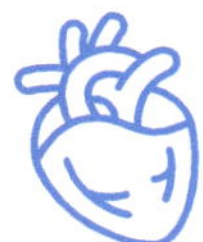

BLOOD PRESSURE (RISK FACTOR – HYPERTENSION)

To monitor your own blood pressure, request that your primary care provider (PCP) submit a prescription for an automatic, brachial (bicep, upper arm, above the elbow) blood pressure monitor at your pharmacy to be paid for by your health insurance. Unfortunately, some medical plans do not cover blood pressure monitors and increasingly too many people in underserved communities have inadequate or no health insurance. If you are unable to obtain a blood pressure monitor from your health insurance, consider purchasing one independently if you have the resources. It is an important investment in your health when feasible. If you cannot obtain a

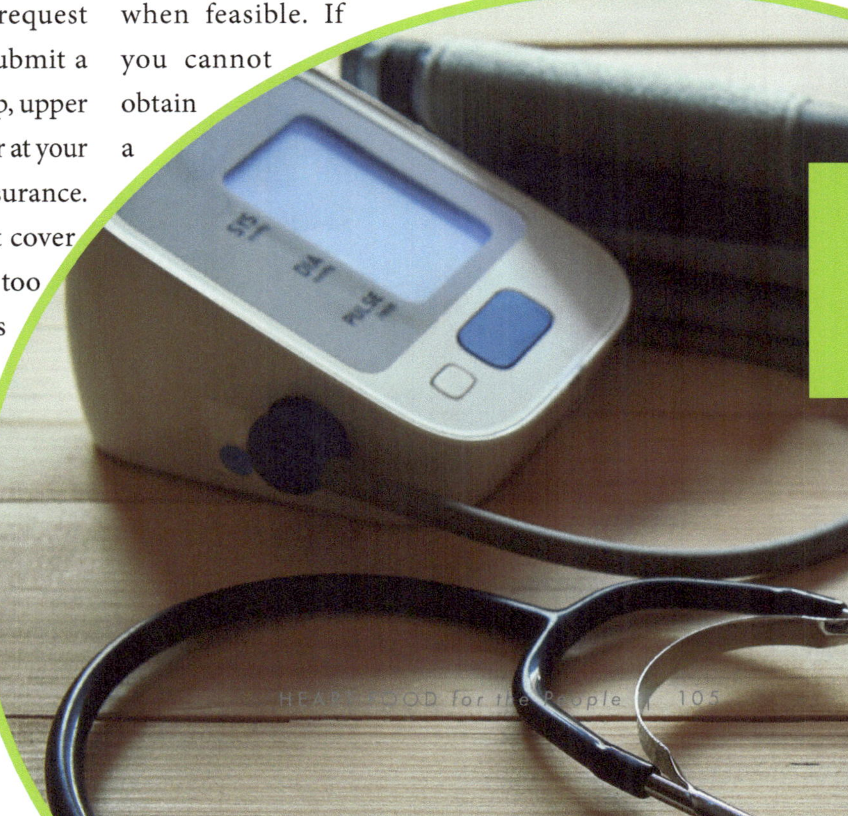

blood pressure monitor, many neighborhood pharmacies have this resource available for public use. Once you have access to a blood pressure monitor, obtain an initial blood pressure measurement and record it in a log you will use to monitor all your cardiovascular disease risk factors.

To ensure you measure your blood pressure correctly always sit quietly in a chair for five minutes before taking your pressure, sit straight up with your back against the chair, keep both feet on the floor, rest your arm on a flat surface (table, chair armrest), and follow the manufacturer's instructions for your specific blood pressure monitor carefully. For additional directions to accurately measure and monitor your blood pressure at home consult the following link:

https://www.heart.org/en/health-topics/high-blood-pressure/understanding-blood-pressure-readings/monitoring-your-blood-pressure-at-home

If your systolic blood pressure (top number) is less than 120mmHg and diastolic blood pressure (bottom number) is less than 80mmHg, you have normal blood pressure. Continue your current Health Empowerment strategy and monitor your blood pressure every six months.

If your systolic blood pressure is between 120 – 129mmHg and diastolic blood pressure is less than 80mmHg you have elevated blood pressure. Intensify your Health Empowerment strategy with a specific focus on reduced salt intake, reduced saturated fat intake, increased fiber intake, and increased frequency and duration of regular cardiac exercise. In addition, monitor your blood pressure every three months.

If your systolic blood pressure is equal to or above 130mmHg or your diastolic blood pressure is equal to or above 80mmHg, you have hypertension. Intensify your Health Empowerment strategy with a specific focus on reduced salt intake, reduced saturated fat intake, increased fiber intake, and increased frequency and duration of regular cardiac exercise. Also, speak to your primary care provider about additional strategies to lower your blood pressure. In addition, monitor your blood pressure every month.

Be sure to keep a written or digital log of your blood pressure and measure this risk factor based on the schedule above after obtaining an initial value.

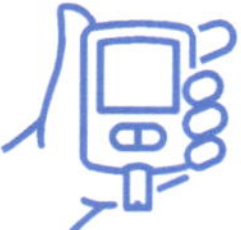

BLOOD GLUCOSE (RISK FACTOR – DIABETES)

To monitor your blood glucose, request that your primary care provider order an initial **HEMOGLOBIN A1C (HA1C) BLOOD TEST.** Access a digital record of the test results or ask your PCP to give you a printed copy of the test if online access is not possible. Document your initial HA1C in the same log you monitor your blood pressure.

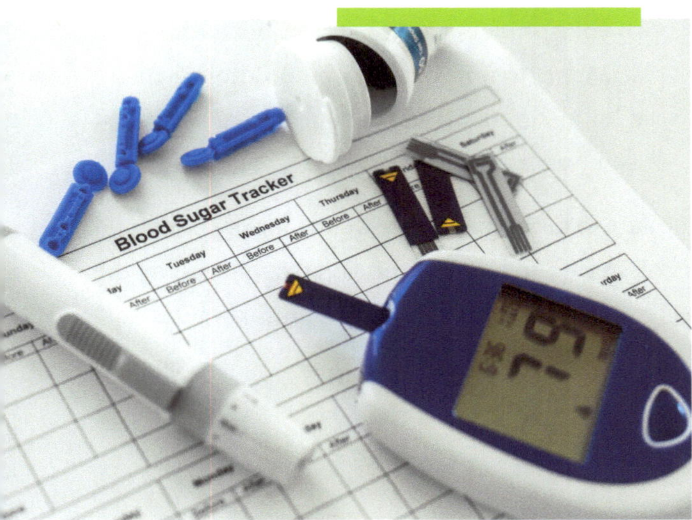

If your HA1C is less than 5.7%, you have a normal blood glucose level. Continue your current Health Empowerment strategy and monitor your HA1C annually.

If your HA1C is between 5.7 – 6.4%, you have pre-diabetes. Intensify your Health Empowerment strategy with a specific focus on reduced processed sugar intake, reduced simple and refined carbohydrate intake, increased fiber intake, and increased frequency and duration of regular cardiac exercise. Also, speak to your primary care provider about additional strategies to lower your blood glucose. In addition, obtain an HA1C blood test every six months

If your HA1C is greater than 6.4% you have diabetes. Intensify your Health Empowerment strategy with a specific focus on reduced pr°ocessed sugar intake, reduced simple and refined carbohydrate intake, increased fiber intake, and increased frequency and duration of regular cardiac exercise. Also, speak to your primary care provider about additional strategies to lower your blood glucose and request a consultation with a diabetes specialist – an Endocrinologist. In addition, obtain an HA1C blood test every three months

Be sure to keep a written or digital log of your blood glucose and monitor this risk factor based on the schedule above after obtaining an initial value.

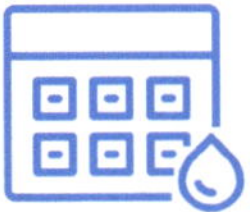

BLOOD CHOLESTEROL (RISK FACTOR – DYSLIPIDEMIA)

To monitor your blood cholesterol, request that your primary care provider order an initial **FASTING LIPID PANEL BLOOD TEST** to include both low-density lipoprotein LDL (bad) cholesterol and high-density lipoprotein HDL (good) cholesterol. Access a digital record of the test results or ask your PCP to give you a printed copy of the test if online access is not possible. Document your initial LDL (bad) and HDL (good) cholesterol in the same log you monitor your blood pressure and blood glucose.

If your LDL cholesterol is less than 70mg/dl and your HDL cholesterol is greater than 50mg/dl you have normal blood cholesterol levels. Continue your current Health Empowerment strategy and monitor your blood cholesterol annually.

Be sure to keep a written or digital log of your blood cholesterol and monitor this risk factor based on the schedule above after obtaining an initial value.

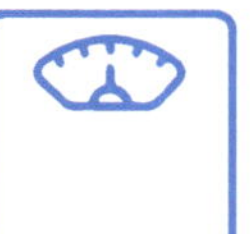

BODY WEIGHT (RISK FACTOR – OBESITY)

To monitor your body weight, use your smartphone or home computer to search for and access a **Body Mass Index (BMI)** calculator on the Internet. Enter your height and most recent weight as instructed and the calculator will provide you with a BMI measurement. Document your initial BMI in the same log you monitor your blood pressure, blood glucose, and blood cholesterol.

If your BMI is between 18.5 to 24.9kg/m2, you have normal body weight. Continue your current Health Empowerment strategy and monitor your BMI every six months

If your BMI is between 25.0 and 29.9kg/m2, you have overweight. Intensify your Health Empowerment strategy with a specific focus on reduced processed sugar intake, reduced simple and refined carbohydrate intake, reduced saturated fat intake, increased fiber intake, and increased frequency and duration of regular cardiac exercise. In addition, calculate your BMI every six months

If your BMI is equal to or greater than 30kg/m2 you have obesity. Intensify your Health Empowerment strategy with a specific focus on reduced processed sugar intake, reduced simple and refined carbohydrate intake, reduced saturated fat intake, increased fiber intake, and increased frequency and duration of regular cardiac exercise. Also, speak to your primary care provider about additional strategies to lower your BMI. In addition, calculate your BMI every three months

Be sure to keep a written or digital log of your BMI and monitor this risk factor based on the schedule above after obtaining an initial value.

A BMI less than 18.5kg/m2 is considered underweight and requires medical attention from your primary care provider

NICOTINE USE (RISK FACTOR – NICOTINE DEPENDENCE)

The goal for the use of nicotine products (cigarettes, vaping, chewing) is always **ZERO**. Because of excessive targeting, marketing, and promotion in underserved communities, combined with the addictive chemicals in nicotine products, this can be an extremely challenging risk factor to manage. However, because it involves the use of an external product it is also the most modifiable and preventable risk factor, and given the significantly increased incidence and prevalence of cardiovascular diseases associated with nicotine dependence, you must make every effort to quit smoking.

If you currently use any nicotine products, immediately implement a self-directed smoking cessation strategy that includes choosing a quit date of personal significance in the near future (3-4 months), gradual reduction of tobacco use leading up to the quit date, and the acquisition and use of nicotine replacement products as instructed by your local Department of Health (nicotine patches, gum, lozenges). Also, speak to your primary care provider about additional strategies for nicotine cessation. (Refer to earlier Nicotine Dependence Section)

Independently monitoring the risk factors that lead to cardiovascular diseases and knowing your goals will enable you to optimize your Health Empowerment strategy, promote wellness, prevent cardiovascular diseases, and live longer and live better.

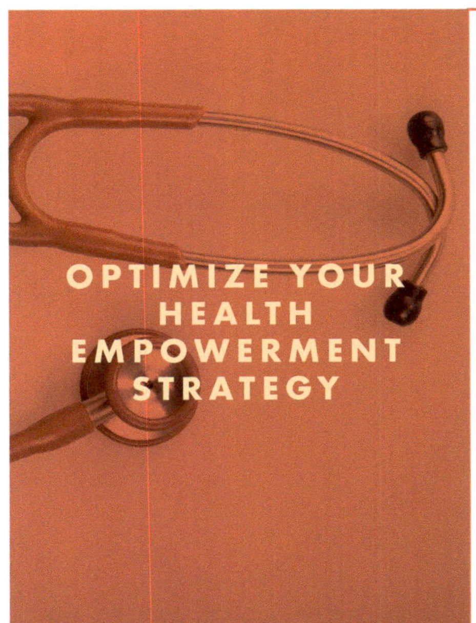

BLOOD PRESSURE GOAL – systolic (top number) less than 120mmHg / diastolic (bottom number) less than 80mmHg

BLOOD GLUCOSE GOAL – Hemoglobin A1C (HA1C) less than 5.7%

BLOOD CHOLESTEROL GOAL – LDL (bad) cholesterol less than 70mg/dl / HDL (good) cholesterol greater than 50mg/dl

BODY WEIGHT GOAL – Body Mass Index (BMI) between 18.5 and 24.9kg/m2

NICOTINE USE GOAL – ZERO

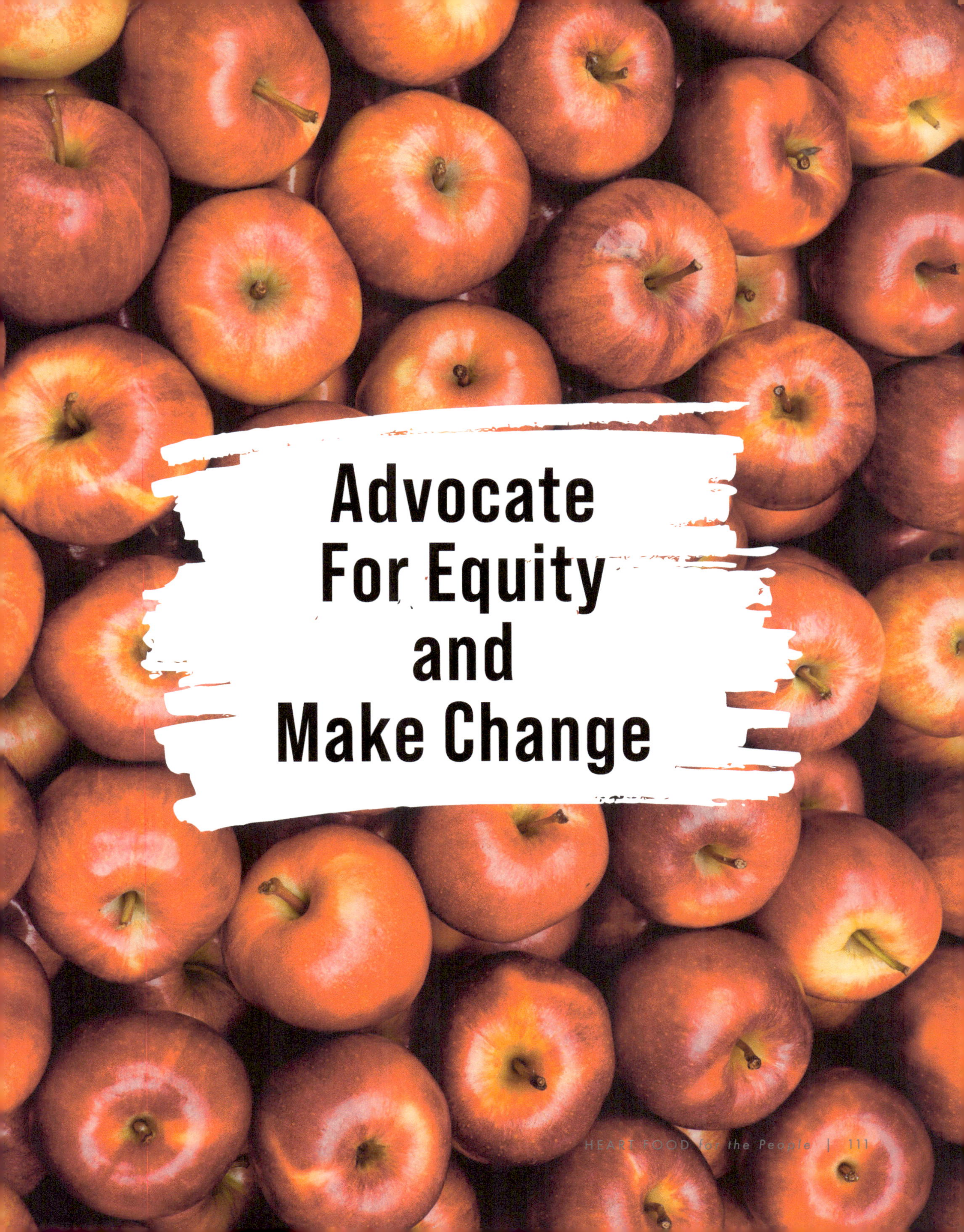
Advocate
For Equity
and
Make Change

ADVOCATE FOR EQUITY AND MAKE CHANGE

The escalating medical system crisis, historical and current economic, political, social, and environmental injustices, and exploitative commercial practices imposed by profiteering corporations, all perpetuate the significant healthcare disparities and inequities that severely impact underserved communities. The result is persistently increased morbidity and mortality, decreased longevity, and diminished quality of physical and mental health.

Health Empowerment is an absolutely imperative reality to ensure underserved communities overcome these lethal challenges, promote wellness, prevent cardiovascular diseases, and live longer and live better. Until healthcare is a universally guaranteed basic human right and everyone has the resources they need to maximize their physical and mental potential we must do everything necessary to empower ourselves.

HEART FOOD *for the People* is a blueprint for this process and provides a detailed strategy for your journey to optimal health, but it is just the beginning. During your unique Health Empowerment journey, you will encounter systemic injustices that limit your ability to protect your life and the lives of the people you love and care about. The systemic injustices adversely affecting underserved communities are profound and include structural racism, generational poverty, residential segregation, land theft, regressive immigration policies, disenfranchisement, and wage suppression. Collectively these injustices entrench healthcare disparities and inequities in underserved communities and make living a healthy life extremely challenging.

Always transform these personal challenges into a movement to advocate for equity. When food deserts, food insecurity, excessive marketing of unhealthy ultra-processed food and nicotine products, limited open space to exercise, health insurance costs, and inadequate access to quality, timely medical care prevent you from living your healthiest life, take immediate action to make meaningful change. Health inequity can only be overcome through radical and revolutionary changes in our society and medical system, including a federal living wage, reparations, land back, plurinational policies, humane and just immigration laws, universal single-payer healthcare, expansion of community-based healthcare centers in every population, and a publicly subsidized focus on preventive health for every community. Contact the health activists, progressive healthcare providers, and grassroots organizations in your community fighting for social justice and health equity and join them in the struggle.

In every underserved community, there are dedicated and committed organizers engaged in the crucial and essential movement for fundamental change. Research and locate them online, through social media, and get involved. The ultimate goal of your individual Health Empowerment journey is to create a reality where health equity is the truth for everyone.

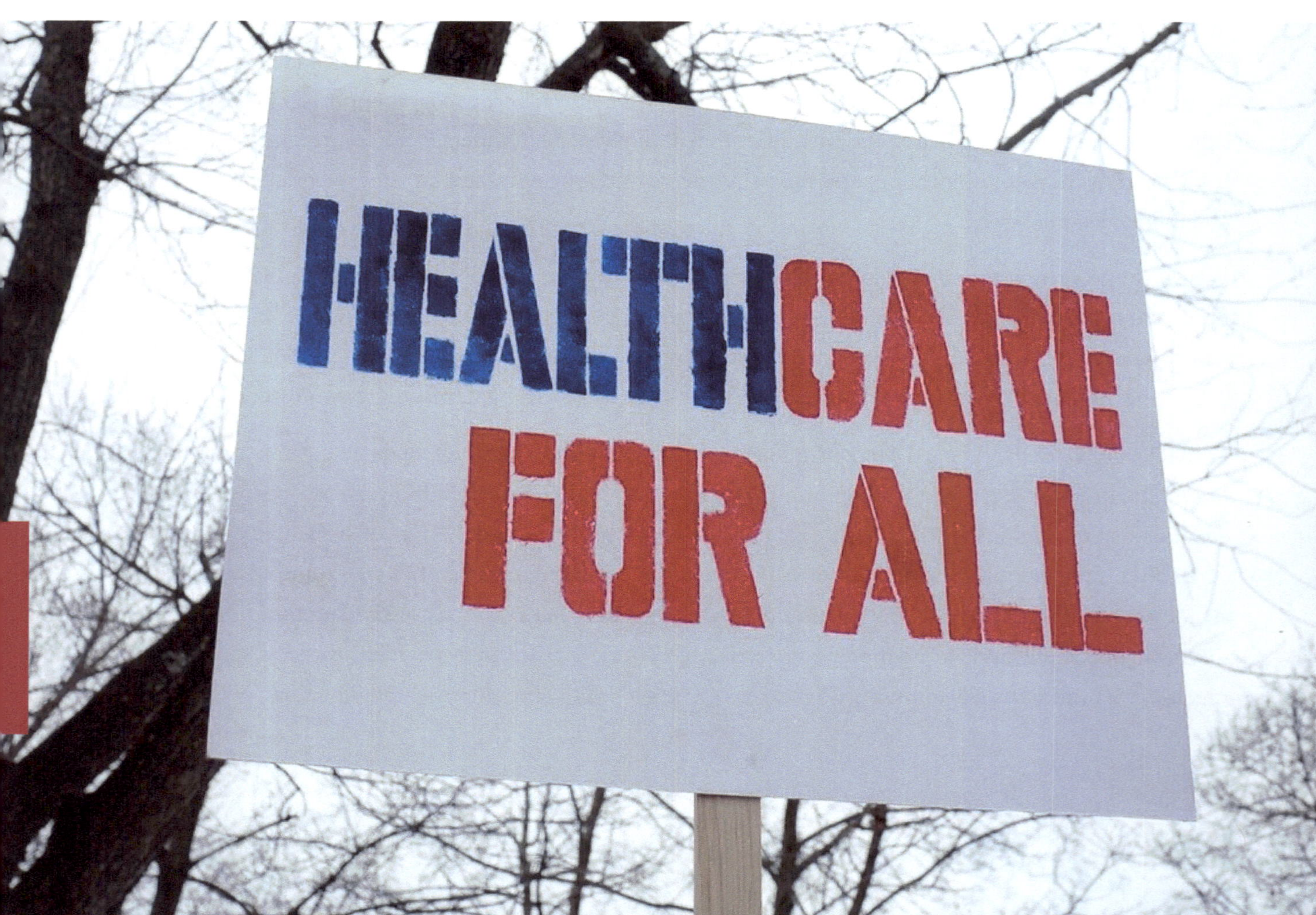

Contact the following grassroots community-based organizations to learn how you can be directly involved in your community's fight for social justice and health equity:

https://www.medicare4all.org

https://www.populardemocracy.org/campaign/organizing-healthcare-justice

https://www.peoplesaction.org/campaigns/health-care-for-all

https://www.reachcoalition.org

https://www.healthcare-now.org

EVIDENCE-BASED SOURCES

The information and strategies in HEART FOOD *for the People* include evidence-based research from the following sources:

American Heart Association

American College of Cardiology

The New England Journal of Medicine

Centers for Disease Control

National Heart, Lung, and Blood Institute

Harvard T.H. Chan School of Public Health – Healthy Living Guide 2023 / 2024

United States Preventive Service Task Force

American Journal of Public Health

International Journal of Food Properties

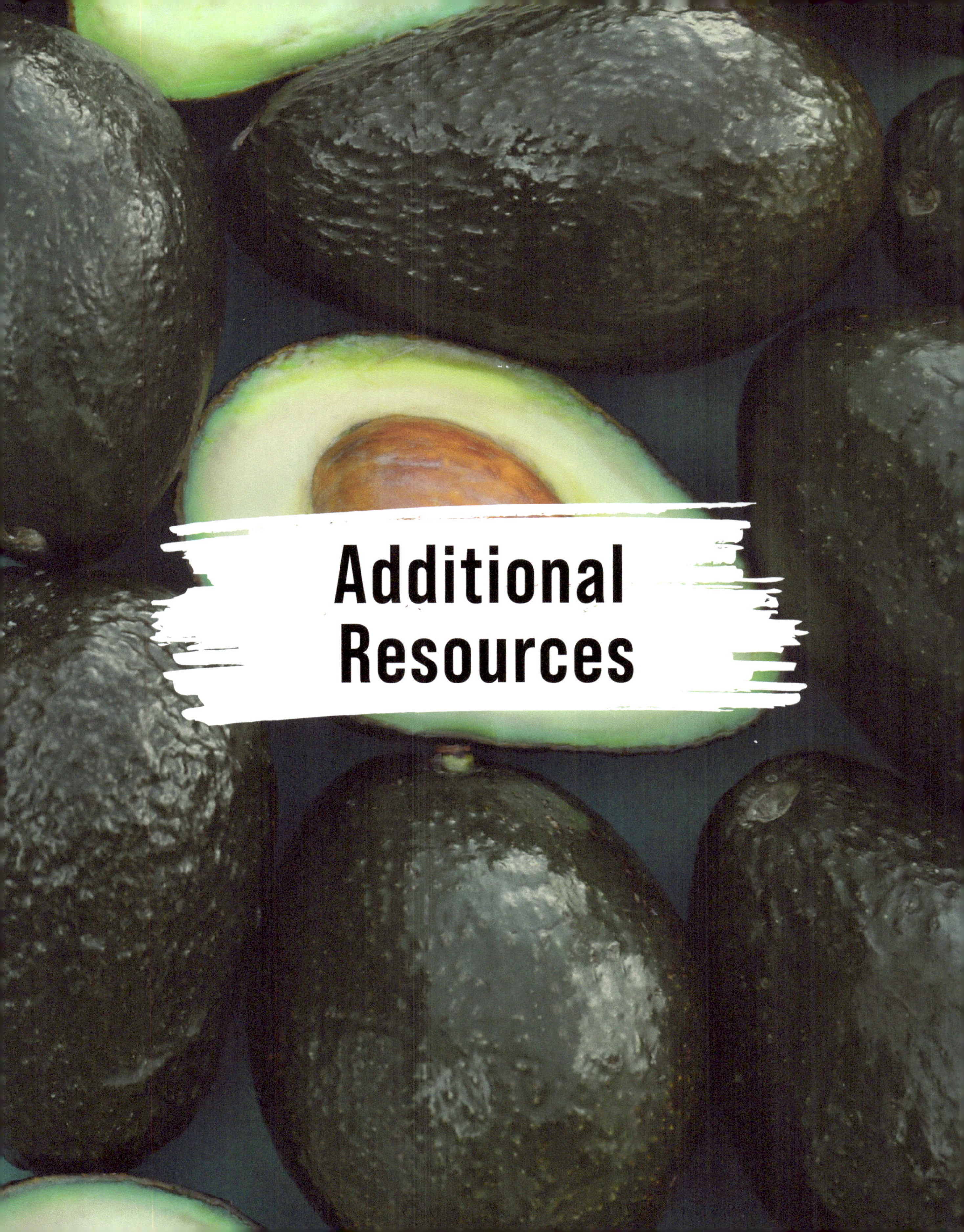

Additional
Resources

ADDITIONAL RESOURCES

Implementing your unique Health Empowerment journey after following the strategies in HEART FOOD *for the People* is a challenging process that will require creativity and innovation.

Below are community-based resources and links for more information that you may find helpful on your journey to optimal health:

FOOD ASSISTANCE

Food insecurity and food deserts make implementing a Health Empowerment strategy challenging in underserved communities by limiting access to nutritious and healthy food. If you need assistance securing heart-healthy food in your community please contact the following organizations and share them with your family and friends:

> https://www.invisiblehandsdeliver.org
> https://www.fullcart.org
> https://www.nutrition.gov/topics/food-security-and-access/
> food-assistance-programs
> https://www.frac.org/programs

THE VEGAN OPTION

Clinical research studies continue to demonstrate the cardiovascular benefits of a strictly plant-based diet that eliminates all foods from animals. In addition, basic science studies continue to reveal the environmental benefits of reducing our cultivation and consumption of animal-based foods. These benefits are particularly important for underserved communities that are disproportionally affected by climate change and global warming because of environmental injustices. Explore the following links if you are interested in researching and starting a vegan nutrition plan as part of your Health Empowerment strategy and share them with your family and friends:

> https://www.vegansociety.com/go-vegan
> https://www.ilovevegan.com/resources/transitioning-to-a-vegan-lifestyle

Farmer's markets and community gardens can often provide free or low-cost, nutritious, and heart-healthy foods not available in local supermarkets and grocery stores. In addition, the organizers of these invaluable resources are often community-based health activists committed to your Health Empowerment and working to secure health equity for everyone. Explore the following links if you are interested in incorporating foods from farmer's markets and community gardens into your Health Empowerment nutrition plan and share them with your family and friends:

https://www.localharvest.org

https://www.communitygarden.org

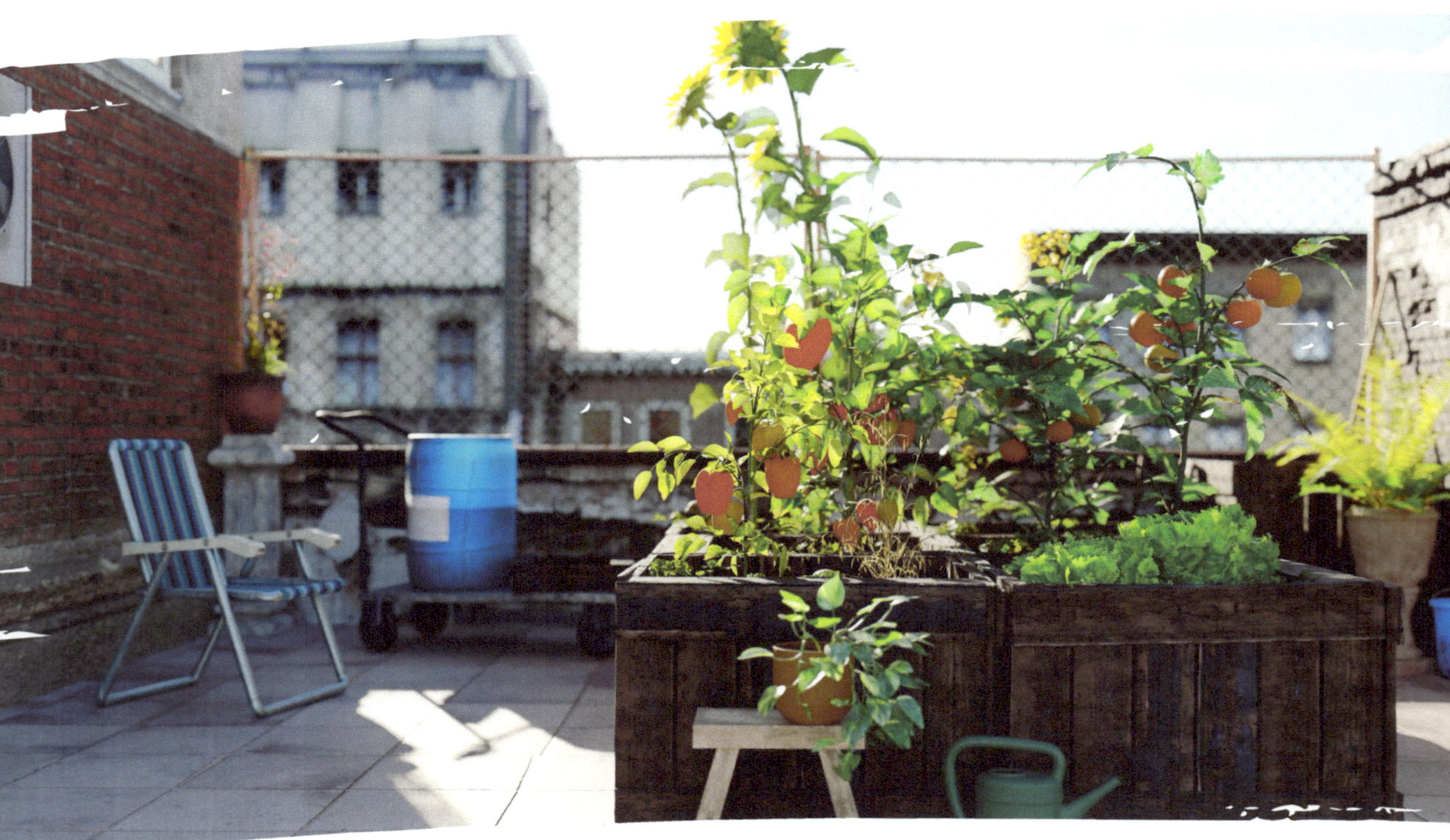

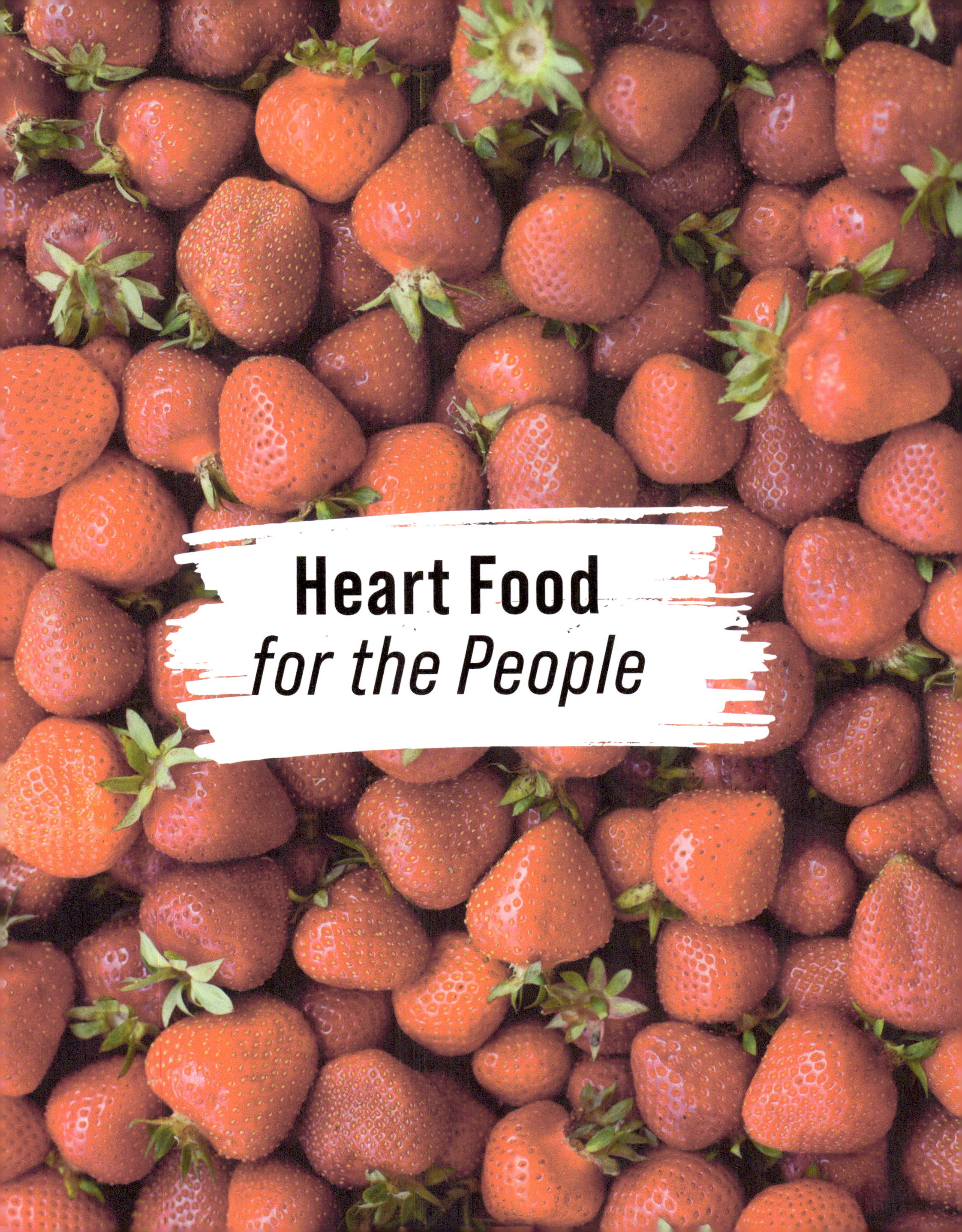
Heart Food
for the People

9 7 9 8 3 3 0 3 3 4 7 2 8